IS *Gwyneth* PALTROW WRONG ABOUT Everything?

HOW THE FAMOUS SELL US ELIXIRS OF HEALTH, BEAUTY & *Happiness*

TIMOTHY CAULFIELD

BEACON PRESS
BOSTON

BEACON PRESS
Boston, Massachusetts
www.beacon.org

Beacon Press books
are published under the auspices of
the Unitarian Universalist Association of Congregations.

22 21 20 19   8 7 6 5 4 3 2

This book is printed on acid-free paper that meets the uncoated paper
ANSI/NISO specifications for permanence as revised in 1992.

Text design and composition by Kim Arney

An early version of my experience with the Clean Cleanse appeared in
Eighteen Bridges (Winter 2013), and an early version of the gluten-free
analysis appeared as "Gluten-Free: Why You Shouldn't Listen
to Miley and Gwyneth," *Toronto Star*, October 18, 2013.

Library of Congress Cataloging-in-Publication Data
Caulfield, Timothy A.
Is Gwyneth Paltrow wrong about everything? : how the famous sell us
elixirs of health, beauty & happiness / Timothy Caulfield.
    pages   cm
Includes bibliographical references and index.
ISBN 978-0-8070-3970-0 (paperback) — ISBN 978-0-8070-5749-0 (ebook)
    1. Quacks and quackery. 2. Celebrities—Health and hygiene.
3. Communication in medicine. 4. Disinformation. 5. Health products.
        6. Popular culture. I. Title.
            R730.C375 2015
            613.2—dc23
            2014041726

For the superstars in my life:
Adam, Alison, Jane, Michael, and Joanne

ABOUT THE AUTHOR

Timothy Caulfield is a Canada Research Chair in Health Law and Policy, a professor in the Faculty of Law and the School of Public Health at the University of Alberta, and research director of the Health Law Institute at the University of Alberta. Over the past several years he has been involved in a variety of interdisciplinary research endeavors that have allowed him to publish over three hundred academic articles. He is a fellow of the Trudeau Foundation and the principal investigator for a number of large interdisciplinary projects that explore the ethical, legal, and health policy issues associated with a range of topics, including stem cell research, genetics, patient safety, the prevention of chronic disease, obesity policy, the commercialization of research, complementary and alternative medicine, and access to health care. Professor Caulfield is and has been involved with a number of national and international policy and research ethics committees. He has won numerous academic awards and is a fellow of the Royal Society of Canada and the Canadian Academy of Health Sciences. He writes frequently for the popular press and is the author of *The Cure for Everything: Untangling Twisted Messages About Health, Fitness, and Happiness.*

Praise for *The Cure for Everything*

"[Caulfield] thinks with an academic's rigor and precision and knows the health maintenance territory inside out. Mr. Caulfield is at his breezy best in discussions of exercise and diet, both of which he approaches with a certain swagger. . . . Caulfield muses at amusing and instructive length on the exact definition of fitness—the bizarre, science-free equivalency the modern aesthetic has established between fitness and sexy abs—and the depressingly well-validated fact that the older you get, the more running it takes to stay in exactly the same place."

—Abigail Zuger, MD, *The New York Times*

CONTENTS

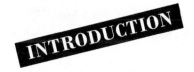

Idol Dreams

"Damn, I shouldn't have slept so long" is my first thought when I see the size of the line, which is already the width of a boxcar and the length of an aircraft carrier. It is early in the morning and cold. Many of my line mates have blankets and a diminishing food supply. It is clear they have been here for a very long time.

The people in the line come in three categories: teenager, young adult, and parent. The last category is, by far, the smallest. And its members are invariably attached to someone from the first category. This makes me an oddball. As far as I can tell, I am the only solo middle-aged man. I try to look confident and purposeful, as if I am here for some specific and important reason, but I am sure I look mostly awkward and out of place.

"What are you doing here?" a young woman asks me through a big friendly smile. She is dressed in an outfit that gives her the appearance of someone who just walked off the set of a Mötley Crüe video, circa 1987.

I want to say, "Making a complete fool of myself," especially since I am in serious need of caffeine and do not feel particularly chatty. Instead I offer an ambiguous "I'm not really sure."

"What are your goals?" I ask the woman, who goes by the not-uncool moniker Shakespeare Sunday.

"I want to make it. And this seems a good place to start," she replies. "*American Idol* needs a rock star!" All the people within earshot of this last comment raise their arms and let out a loud "*Wooooooo!*" It is as if this group of strangers has rehearsed the moment, which ends in high-fives and fist bumps.

Ms. Sunday hands me her smartphone and invites me to listen to a recording of her work, which is much better than I expected—though I am not sure what I expected. Before the song finishes, Ms. Sunday (I just can't bring myself to call her Shakespeare) notices a commotion down the line and abruptly ends our exchange. She pushes toward the edge of the line, grooming herself as she goes. Ms. Sunday has spotted a TV camera.

A man with a microphone is interviewing people in the line, asking them about their hometown, what makes them special, and, of course, if they are the next winner of *American Idol*. As the camera crew tracks the lineup, a wave of preening and posing moves with it. The criteria for selection as an interviewee seem straightforward: those selected are attractive and/or have something distinctive about their appearance. My new friend, Ms. Sunday, is among the chosen. She satisfies both requirements but mostly the latter.

I am not (at least currently) a singer, and I do not have any plans to become one. My voice is terrible. Fortunately, my future does not depend on it. I am a university professor who has spent the last twenty years researching and writing about the health policy implications of things like genetics, stem cell research, obesity, health care reform, and personalized medicine. So what the heck am I doing at an *American Idol* audition? Well, I hope to audition! And why do I want to audition? Because I want to learn more about, and get as close as I can to, the phenomenon of celebrity. And nothing represents celebrity culture better than *American Idol*.

During the past few decades, celebrity culture's grip on our society has tightened. This is a truism. I don't need to convince anyone that we live in the age of celebrity. Yes, celebrities have been part of the cultural landscape for most of human history. From Alexander the Great to Lord Byron, we have always been fascinated with the famous. But never has celebrity culture played such a dominant role in so many aspects of our lives. It has a measurable influence on individual health-care decisions, the things we do to stay healthy, how we view ourselves physically, the material goods we want to possess, and our future career aspirations. Whether we like it or not, celebrity culture has a profound impact on our world, framing how we think about important issues and even influencing how we view our place in the universe. But this is not a book *about* celebrity culture—there are many interesting and thoughtful treatises on the nature and causes of our obsession with famous people. Rather, in this book I analyze and debunk the messages and promises—implicit and explicit—that flow from the celebrity realm, be they about health, diet, beauty, our ambitions, or what is supposed to make us happy.

Many writers have proposed definitions of celebrity culture. For this book I am interested in our preoccupation with, and the value we attach to, celebrity lifestyles and to celebrities themselves—whether in the realm of movies, music, or sports—and all the industries and social structures that create and sustain them. Celebrity culture is often blamed for dumbing down our social discourse, but less has been said about how it is a source of misinformation. Indeed, celebrity culture has emerged as one of the most significant and influential sources of pseudoscientific blather. It fills our cultural landscape with notions ranging from those that are patently absurd and widely mocked (such as Simon Cowell's hiring of a psychic "house healer" to exorcise his home of "negative energy") to those that gain substantial social traction and market appeal. The popularity of juicing, cleanses, detox diets, weird exercise routines, and a boatload of beauty and antiaging products and practices can be linked directly to celebrity endorsements. Think, for example, of Kate Perry's and Hilary Swank's advocacy of vitamins, Gwyneth Paltrow's enthusiasm for colon cleanses and a gluten-free diet, Jennifer Aniston's ballyhooed belief in water cures, or just about every celebrity's advice on how to lose weight.

Looking at these health and well-being issues through the lens of celebrity culture may seem frivolous. But we should not underestimate the impact celebrities can have on our preferences and attitudes—which is, of course, why they are so frequently paid millions of dollars by advertisers to move product. Specific examples abound. Angelina Jolie's revelation that genetic testing precipitated her decision to have a preventative mastectomy resulted in an immediate increase in demand for both genetic testing and preventative mastectomies. Similarly, and perhaps more troubling, images of celebrities smoking—in film, on TV shows, and in magazines—are linked to an increase in cigarette consumption. The celebrity trend for using beautifying and rejuvenating vitamin intravenous therapy has reportedly caused a shortage of critical medical supplies. Ill-informed celebrity statements about the alleged risks associated with vaccines (most notably by Jenny McCarthy) have adversely impacted public dialog about the value of vaccines. And, most disturbingly, reports of celebrity suicides are associated with an increase in suicide in the general public. I could go on and on and on.

Some have suggested that humans are evolutionarily wired to follow and perhaps be influenced by people they look up to. Many species, including other primates, carefully watch dominant individuals within their group. Evolutionary psychologists have speculated that this tendency evolved as part of a package of innate predispositions that allow humans to learn from successful role models. The process happens unconsciously. While this propensity may have helped prehistoric hunter-gatherers to acquire useful bits of knowledge and skill, in the context of modern society, following Gwyneth Paltrow's health advice or coveting Kim Kardashian's life provides little benefit. In fact, in the pages that follow I will argue that this propensity has emerged as one of our society's most pernicious forces, contributing to, among other things, poor health decisions, wasted investments in useless beauty and fitness products, a decreased understanding of how science works, and increased dissatisfaction with our appearance and perhaps our lives.

Of course, the impact of celebrity culture reaches well beyond the areas of health and beauty. Increasingly, people see becoming a celebrity or obtaining a celebrity lifestyle as a reasonable and obtainable life goal. Even President Barack Obama has commented on the trend. In a 2013 interview he suggested that the constant exposure to "the lifestyles of the rich and famous" has caused "a shift in culture." In the past "kids weren't monitoring every day what Kim Kardashian was wearing, or where Kanye West was going on vacation, and thinking that somehow that was the mark of success," Obama said. These comments are both unusual (how many times has the leader of the free world taken time to speculate about the social impact of a reality TV star?) and correct.

Ample evidence supports Obama's observations. Survey research from the United States has revealed that becoming famous is now viewed as a key part of the American dream. And numerous studies have found that becoming a celebrity—or gaining success in a celebrity-oriented profession such as singing, acting, or sports—has emerged as the primary aspiration of a substantial segment of the population. Social media have played a significant role in this development, by bringing celebrities closer to the public and multiplying the opportunities to make social comparisons. The celebrity life seems real, awesome, and accessible. One study, published in 2013, found that social media interactions with celebrities, particularly through Twitter, allow fans to feel that they have an "authentic" relationship with their idols. Fans have the sense, rightly or not, that the interactions are real, which in turn leads them to become more "involved and invested in celebrities' lives."

The central goal of this book is simple: to get to the truth about the claims that flow from celebrity culture, be they about the diets that purport to make us thin, the antiaging products that will keep us forever youthful and wrinkle free, or the actions that we are told we should take, such as auditioning for *American Idol*, to propel us into the realm of celebrity. I seek to separate sense from nonsense and provide usable and evidence-informed advice about the strategies that actually work and those that are a complete waste of money and time. I will look at everything from vitamins, organic food, and gluten-free diets to the odds of making it big as an actor, musician, or professional athlete. I will also explore the impact of celebrity culture on things like body image, the use of cosmetic surgery, and unhealthy behaviors, such as binge dieting and sunbathing. I also will examine what it is like to be a celebrity and the social and biological forces that seem to compel many of us to "reach for the stars."

To this end I have deployed a range of traditional scholarly methods, including analyzing the best available scientific data and interviewing renowned academic and clinical experts. But I also tried to gain an understanding of various aspects of the celebrity universe and its social impact by interacting with actors, musicians, and even porn stars. To put my research in context, I tried celebrity-recommended beauty routines and diets. I signed on with a modeling agency and went to a modeling competition in New York. And I have tried to immerse myself in the celebrity-oriented media. For example, I followed celebrity Twitter feeds, read gossip blogs, and forced myself to read every issue—cover to cover—of the world's most popular celebrity-oriented publication, *People*, for an entire year. The book is organized into two sections, one focusing on the illusion of celebrity authority and one on the illusion that one can become a celebrity. These sections explore the cumulative effect of three celebrity-driven illusions: that celebrity culture embodies a real, achievable, and desirable ideal of health and beauty and confers on celebrities the authority to impart health and beauty advice; that the status of celebrity can (and should) be achieved by anyone who dreams big, works hard, or believes in him or herself with sufficient intensity (an illusion I witnessed firsthand at the *American Idol* audition and one that is central to the role celebrity culture plays in our lives); and, finally, that celebrities lead the happiest, most desirable, most fulfilled lives.

A FEW WORDS about tone: I do not mean to mock those who enjoy popular culture or follow celebrities. On the contrary, I *love* celebrity culture. I always have. Indeed, my interest in celebrity culture is one reason I wanted to write this book. When I play Trivial Pursuit, the only questions I can reliably answer are the ones from the entertainment category. Each award season, without any effort, I somehow become aware of all the nominees for the Golden Globes, the Grammys, and, of course, the Oscars. I even have a vague knowledge of the celebrities in the running for a People's Choice Award. It's as if the names of the nominees are implanted in my brain as I sleep. I probably know more about Pamela Anderson and Gwyneth Paltrow than about Albert Einstein, Albert Camus, or, for that matter, Albert, my neighbor. So if you love and follow celebrity culture, this book is for you.

I am also not going to try to deny or minimize the power of celebrity. Being near the famous does create an odd, unquantifiable electricity. I felt it myself when, in order to get into the swing of things, I attended the Hollywood premiere of the movie *This Is the End*, starring James Franco, Seth Rogen, Jonah Hill, and Emma Watson. I don't mean that I was invited to attend the premiere or to interview the stars. No, I stood outside the theater with hordes of screaming fans waiting for the stars to be delivered in big black limos. At first I tried to fool myself into believing that I was there as an academic, an impartial observer. I was Jane Goodall in the Hollywood jungle. But as each limo pulled up I got progressively more into it, standing on my tippy toes to see who would emerge from the vehicle.

"Is that James?" I asked no one in particular. It was not. I sighed along with my neighbors. "Oh! It's nobody!"

We all hoped the stars would come to our corner of the line. So we would yell things like "Emma! Emma! Over here!" It didn't work. Pencil-thin Emma Watson waved in our direction but did not stop. But normal-size Seth Rogen did. Indeed, I swear that Seth and I had a moment, locking eyes in a kind of friendly, if silent, exchange.

"Seth seems like a nice guy," I said to the guy standing next to me. How the hell would I know that? And why did I want to tell a stranger?

So it's true: celebrities have the capacity to cast a spell on us all. Celebrity culture really is, as the research tells us, a tremendously powerful force. Given this reality, this book is also relevant for those of you who hate celebrity culture—and I know you are out there because I heard from many of you while I was writing it. If you're looking for further reason to be skeptical of celebrity culture and its impact on our society, the pages that follow will provide you with an abundance of science-informed ammunition.

# # #

SHOWS LIKE *AMERICAN IDOL* leverage this fascination with celebrities and our desire to reap the rewards of celebrity status. Indeed, the promise of becoming a celebrity is the unspoken reward for appearing on the show— hence my decision to start my journey at an *American Idol* audition.

The massive line of wannabes moves much faster than I expect. *American Idol* is an efficient machine, processing participants as a factory farm processes chickens. Today is only the registration phase. If I satisfy some basic criteria, I will get a wristband that allows me to audition tomorrow morning.

The rules state that I must be an American citizen. Check. A person must not have done well on a previous *American Idol* season. Check. I must not have a current recording contract. Check. I must not have a close personal or family relationship with the company that owns *American Idol*. Check. And I must be between the ages of fifteen and twenty-eight. OK, this last requirement could be a challenge.

Still, I have taken this audition seriously. If given the opportunity, I intend to sing "Lost in the Supermarket," by the Clash. In the past few weeks I have rehearsed a slightly jazzy version of the song in front of my kids, who invariably give me severe Simon Cowell–ish feedback: "Terrible." "Out of tune." "What key was that?" But despite their harsh reviews, I feel that I've prepared a unique and only marginally embarrassing audition piece. I am ready for my chance!

All the *American Idol* employees wear pale blue T-shirts embossed with the show's logo and headsets attached to walkie-talkie devices. One escorts me to a table where a woman will decide if I can move on to the next phase of the competition. The woman, who is young enough to be a contestant, looks me up and down, and I can tell by her you-have-got-to-be-kidding smile and the tilt of her head that she has made her decision. But before she can announce her verdict, I launch into a plea.

"Look, I know I am a bit too old," I say quickly.

She grimaces. "A bit?"

"But I really want to do this, and I've got a great song prepared!"

Seeing that I am getting nowhere and fearing that I am going to be tossed out, I relent and tell her about my book project. To my surprise, she seems intrigued. After I make my case to the onsite producer, the *Idol* team agrees to let me come back tomorrow. I can't audition, but I can hang with the contestants. Good enough. My jazzy, punk styling will need to wait for another day.

I return to the *American Idol* auditions the next morning just as the contestants are gathering under a TV camera attached to the end of a massive boom. The camera swings over the crowd, generating screams and the waving of signs informing the world that the holder "Has Got It" and we should "Look No Further" and, of course, that he or she is "the Next American Idol." The scene is repeated again and again as an *Idol* employee with a megaphone calls for more enthusiasm with each pass of the camera.

Currently in its thirteenth season, *American Idol* has developed into a true cultural phenomenon. Tens of thousands of individuals have auditioned for the show. From 2003 to 2011 it was the highest-rated show on TV. Though it has lost momentum over the past few seasons, in 2013 it was still ranked as the seventh-most-watched regularly scheduled program on TV. And its influence has led to the introduction of other reach-for-the-stars-and-become-a-celebrity shows, such as *America's Got Talent*, *The X Factor*, *The Voice*, and *So You Think You Can Dance*.

It's no surprise, then, that so many view *Idol* as a vehicle they can ride to superstardom. As I mingle and chat with the contestants, I hear this theme again and again. "Singing is everything," one teenage girl tells me. She is standing alone at the edge of the crowd, wearing a baggy hoodie and jeans, her long hair obscuring much of her face. She views the show as her best chance at fame and fortune because, as she explains, she has "never had any money." As a child she was abused, so when she becomes a star (she tells this in a matter-of-fact tone that suggests she is certain this will happen), she intends to "help the less fortunate." A weak "good luck" is all I can muster in the face of her puzzling optimism.

I chat with many contestants who have been to multiple auditions. One young woman with bright-red hair has auditioned five times, never making it past the first round. "Just nerves," she explains. Another, a fifteen-year-old who informs me that "this is her dream" and "something she has wanted her whole life," just finished competing on the rival TV show *The X Factor*.

While a few people say their expectations are modest, and are auditioning merely for the experience, the vast majority seem to be swinging for the fences. Big-time fame is the goal. They all tell me that you must "reach for the stars" and "hold onto your dreams" and "continue to believe" and that singing is "the number-one priority in life."

Then a strange thing happens. I look up from my notepad and find a small crowd gathering around me—a tight semicircle of smiling contestants eager to be interviewed. Some are throwing my way bits of biographical information—their age, their experience, and their multiple talents. It occurs to me that they think I am from a reputable newspaper or magazine, but my explanation that I am working on a book project does little to dampen the enthusiasm. Everyone wants to be interviewed. They want exposure. Just when I start to worry that my little scrum might get out of hand, I am saved by none other than Ryan Seacrest.

"Who is ready to change their life today?!" Seacrest screams. "Is the next American Idol here?" Everyone goes berserk.

Seacrest moves through the crowd, a camera crew recording his genial interactions with the contestants. He comes closer and closer to my position. And just when it seems possible that he is going to back into me, I make a fatal mistake. I take out my phone and snap a few pictures. Who can blame me? It's Ryan Seacrest! He is so close, I could touch his perfectly coiffed hair.

A headset-wearing *Idol* employee taps me on the shoulder. "Excuse me," she says, "but you don't belong here."

Part I

The Illusion of
Celebrity Authority

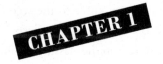

Dieting, Gwyneth, and My Cleanse

Donna Karan and Demi Moore are just two among many celebrities who have raved about the diet regime that just about everyone associates with Gwyneth Paltrow. Indeed, if celebrity endorsements were proof of a product's effectiveness, the Clean Cleanse that Gwyneth is always talking about would be beyond criticism. So it seems to me that the obvious place to start my investigation of the cleanse is in London, home of Gwyneth's booming e-commerce company, Goop. I figure I will ask the employees of Goop about the Gwyneth-inspired cleanse experience before I try it myself. Gwyneth often writes about it in her Goop blogs. She has said, "This thing is amazing," that it "worked wonders," and that it made her feel "pure and happy and much lighter." She has also noted that it is something that she does with the whole "Goop team."

I'd love to feel pure, happy, and lighter. OK, I'm not sure what that would feel like, but it sounds better than I usually feel. Who wouldn't want to feel like that? Given the warm and friendly vibe on the Goop website—it was, after all, to quote the website, "created to celebrate all life's positives"—I am expecting a warm and happy vibe at Goop HQ.

I am mistaken. Apparently, I am not one of life's positives.

I ring the buzzer to request entry to the second-floor office. No response. I try again and then again. Still no response. I implement Plan B. As a courier is buzzed up, I do the classic foot-in-the-door move. I feel like Jason Bourne.

I confidently walk up to the Goop receptionist and give her a friendly hello. She does not say, "May I help you?" or even "Do you have an appointment?" Instead I get a blank Goopless stare. Undaunted, I ask to see someone about the cleanse, trying my best to give the impression that I am here for a prearranged meeting. She looks at me as if I am a homeless man asking for spare change. In other words, she doesn't look at me. She picks up the phone—still not a word to me—to tell someone about my presence in the office. Then I wait. And wait. Just when I start to fear a Goop security guard will appear, doubtless wearing a tasteful Stella McCartney–inspired ensemble, a young woman approaches me. "You're here to talk about the Clean Cleanse?" she says brightly.

Finally! I think. *This is more like it. My dogged journalistic persistence has paid off.* "That's right," I say. "I'd really like to know more about what actually takes place in the cleanse. I want to get some details about the process and the science behind it."

She smiles. "What a good idea."

This is unfolding precisely as I'd hoped it would. "Thank you," I say. "Who would you suggest I speak with?" I imagine Gwyneth herself now cooperating with my investigation.

"I would say Dhru Purohit," says the charming young lady.

I take out my notebook, expecting her to lead me down the hall to the office of said person. "And where would I find him?"

"Santa Monica, I believe." Her smile now is accompanied by an arched eyebrow. "Which is where the Clean Program is based. You know that, right? That they're the company that makes the Clean Cleanse?"

I close my notebook. Jason Bourne did not have to implement Plan B to exit the building.

# # #

AFTER A FEW phone calls and e-mails about my desire to do the cleanse, Dhru Purohit has a kit sent to my house (the usual price is $425). He also invites me to the Santa Monica office to obtain some precleanse advice and to meet the guru himself, Dr. Alejandro Junger.

The building is inconspicuous. It is not the type of structure you would expect for the head office of a wildly successful diet company. The Clean Program has produced several international best-selling books and tens of thousands of Clean Cleanses, which the company website heralds as "the most endorsed, supported and effective cleanse in the world." And yet its offices, just a block off Los Angeles's often-sung-about Santa Monica Boulevard, look like a modest walk-up apartment. "Do they live here?" I wonder as I approach the door. There is no sign announcing the name of the company. There isn't even a nameplate. There is just a buzzer.

But if the building is understated, its occupants are not. When it comes to life's positives, the Goop team in London could learn a thing or two from Dhru Purohit. This guy is fun. He is all energy, enthusiasm, and commitment. "Hey, Tim!" Purohit says with a big, welcoming smile as soon as the door swings open. He invites me into the company's modern work space, which looks more like an open-concept home than a business. No offices, cubicles, or desks in sight—just a large kitchen and several comfy-looking sofas and chairs. Purohit tells me he is "a Sherpa of sorts." He's a guy who "enjoys guiding people and communities through the world of holistic healing and spiritual living." And he believes in the cleanse product the way Napoleon believed in the flexible use of artillery. It may not be easy to implement, but it can change the world.

Dr. Junger is scheduled to arrive in a few minutes, so I take the time to ask Purohit about what I view as the biggest challenge associated with the cleanse: no coffee. "I am a coffee addict," I tell him. "I love coffee. I cannot stress this enough. It is central to my very existence. Are you sure I must give it up?"

"You must give your adrenals a rest," he explains. "And you must remove the dependency. The idea that you need coffee to function, long term, stresses your adrenals. Your adrenals are your energy bank account."

I will hear the word *adrenal*—which, I assume, is a reference to the hormones secreted by the adrenal glands—approximately nine thousand times during my interactions with the Clean Program teams. *Adrenal glands. Adrenal fatigue. Adrenal stress. Adrenal rest.*

Moments later Junger arrives. I will say this about the man: he projects a relaxed energy. He's got his adrenals in check, obviously. His posture is relaxed, his voice is relaxed, and his outfit is relaxed. I'm pretty sure he is wearing hand-knitted slipper shoes. I can see why Gwyneth likes hanging with him. I feel more Zen-like just being in his presence.

Purohit tells Junger about my cleanse plan. "It. Will. Blow. Your. Mind," Junger tells me as he settles into one of the comfy chairs, legs crossed as if he is about to meditate.

Junger is a physician from Uruguay. He is the inventor of the Clean Cleanse and is often described in the popular press as Gwyneth Paltrow's doctor, though "spiritual leader" would probably be more accurate. Indeed, Gwyneth's best-selling cookbook, *It's All Good*, is dedicated to, among others, Junger, whom she describes as "my good friend." The book contains recipes inspired by Junger's diet and health philosophy. In the preface, she credits him, and the Clean Cleanse, with curing her of a variety of ailments, including an intestinal parasite that went undetected by Gwyneth's conventional physicians, the adjustment of her "sky-high" adrenals, and the unclogging of her horribly clogged liver. If you believe Gwyneth, the cleanse reduced her levels of stress and improved her looks. Given all this Gwyneth-attention, it is no surprise that Junger is a bit of a celebrity himself, appearing on programs such as *The Dr. Oz Show*, where Junger provides detoxing and cleansing advice.

He explains to me how the cleanse works and why it is so important. There are many references to detoxification, our body's energy systems, our body's natural ability to heal, the evils of gluten, and, naturally, adrenals. He also compares our world to a dirty fish tank filled with "toxic triggers" such as plastic, pollution, and drugs. "The dirty fish tank is, for us, the city. It is unnatural. The more industrialized, the more chemicalized, the more diseases there are." I am not sure that a medieval serf would agree with his analysis, but I get the idea.

At the risk of sounding unconcerned for other Earth dwellers, I tell him that my biggest concern is whether I can hack it. "I'm worried it's going to be too tough," I tell him, my thoughts centered on the coffee ban. "I don't think I can do it."

"Don't declare something you don't know," Junger says. "Keep an open mind. Go with it. You should be thinking, 'I wonder how this is going to transform me?'"

I AM THREE DAYS into my cleanse, and my family is not impressed. They are ready to cleanse me from their lives. My sanity is questioned, my company avoided. My eating habits are characterized as revolting. And, to add insult to self-inflicted injury, they tell me my breath stinks.

At this stage I do not feel clean or pure or happy. I feel and behave like a miserable bastard. The combination of caffeine withdrawal and hunger pangs has transformed me into a feral beast with a fuse as short as one of Gwyneth's fabulous dresses. (Specifically, I'm thinking of that minimalist number she wore to the opening of her fitness studio in Hollywood. The dress is a Victoria Beckham design, I believe. But the lack of coffee has left me pretty confused, so I can't be sure. Perhaps it was an Alexander Wang.)

You are probably wondering what the cleanse involves. What is the magic formula that will transform me? Here are the basics. For breakfast I suck back a shake made out of a prepackaged powder that looks but does not taste like the chocolate milk mix I loved as a kid. It is neither appetizing nor satisfying. I must use almond or coconut milk because no dairy products are allowed. This concoction is also my evening meal. Every evening. Needless to say, I go to bed hungry. For lunch I can have real food, but the selection is greatly restricted. Apples are OK but not bananas. Lemons yes, oranges no. No raisins. I can have organic chicken and wild fish but no beef or pork. No wheat or gluten, naturally. Sugar is verboten (though the fact that many foods have naturally occurring sugar in them is never addressed by the Clean Program team). No eggs. And, sadly, because I really feel like I could use some, no alcohol. I must also consume a variety of supplements, including a boatload of probiotics.

I showed my colleague, Professor Linda McCarger, a renowned clinical nutritionist and metabolism researcher, the ingredients of the Clean Cleanse shake mix and supplements. "Looks like they are simply trying to remove everything often associated with an allergic response. They seem to be working off the gluten-free, allergy-free trend," is her initial reaction to the information sheet provided by the Clean Program. I was curious about some of the specific ingredients in the chocolaty powder; in general, she saw nothing unique in them. "They have components like rice syrup. But there is nothing special about that. It is just not made from wheat . . . but it is still a sweetener, used by the body like other syrups. No magic."

This spartan, not-magic existence lasts for twenty-one days. I've got seventeen to go. I have serious doubts about whether I can make it. I keep reminding myself that Gwyneth does this on a regular basis. She is tougher than I thought.

CLEANSING, DRIVEN LARGELY by celebrity endorsements, has become an extraordinarily popular trend. It now involves the sale of special detoxifying juices (currently estimated to be a $5 billion market), cleansing programs (such as the one I am on), and colon cleanses (yep, exactly what it sounds like). There is also a baffling array of books on cleansing and detoxification. Here is a far-from-comprehensive list of just the books that have duration as their primary theme, in descending order of urgency: *The One Month Carb Detox*, *The 4-Week Ultimate Body Detox Plan*, *The 21-Day Sugar Detox*, *The 14-Day Detox Diet*, *The 12-Day Detox Guide*, *The 10-Day Detox Diet*, *The 9-Day Liver Detox Diet*, *The 8-Day Detox Breakthrough*, *The 7-Day Detox Miracle*, *The 6-Day Detox Drop*, *The 5-Day Kidney Detox*, *The 4-Day Detox* (not to be confused with the *Detox 4 Women*), *The 3-Day Green Smoothie Detox*, *The Food Combining 2-Day Detox*, and, for those in a real hurry, *The Fast Track One-Day Detox Diet*.

The concept of cleansing and detoxifying rests on the idea that because of all the toxins in the modern world and all the crap we eat, our bodies need to be scrubbed clean. By doing this, or so the theory goes, we will promote natural healing, reduce stress (the adrenals thing), and reset (a word often associated with cleanses) our system. Cleanses are also presented as a way to look healthier and lose weight. For example, Katy Perry told the world, again and again, that she went on a three-month cleanse that included vitamins and supplements in preparation for the photo shoot she did for her July 2013 cover of *Vogue*. This was because, as Perry told Jay Leno on *The Tonight Show*, she "just wanted to be glowing for that cover."

Cleansing and Detoxifying

Let's start with the central idea. Do our bodies need to be detoxified and will cleansing do the trick?

No and no.

Despite the remarkable popularity of the practice, there is absolutely no evidence to support the idea that we need to detoxify our bodies in the manner suggested by the cleansing industry. The proponents of cleansing often sell the idea by using colorful metaphors that make it all seem so darn logical. The manual for the Clean Cleanse puts it this way: "If you don't take out the trash at your house, it will pile up, attract pests, and quickly become a problem. Having daily bowel movements will help make sure that toxins aren't re-absorbed into your system."

Who wants trash and pests in their colon?

Do not be fooled by these rhetorical games. The idea of detoxing is faulty on so many levels that it borders on the absurd. First, the human body has organs, including the kidneys, liver, skin, and colon, that take care of the detoxification process. When you pee, you are detoxifying. Toxins don't build up, waiting to be cleansed by supplements and special foods. (And, just in case you are wondering, you don't reabsorb toxins by not having your regular bowel movement. Sigh.) There is no evidence that we need to assist our detoxifying organs by ingesting specific foods or supplements. As summarized in a 2005 academic article, "Detox Diets Provide Empty Promises": "These approaches are contrary to scientific consensus and medical evidence and are not consistent with the principle that diets should reflect balance, moderation, and variety."

Second, and more important, there is no evidence that the products and diets sold by the cleansing industry—whether juices, supplements, or specific diet regimens—do anything to help clear toxins, parasites, or bad karma in a manner beneficial to our health. There does not appear to be even a single scientific study to back up the theory behind this massive industry. (OK, I found *one* study, published in the *Journal of Chiropractic Medicine*, which involved seven individuals and no comparison group. The methods are so poor that I am not sure it qualifies as a study.) The British Broadcasting Company did a fun and somewhat scientific-ish experiment involving ten "party animal" young adults. Five got a balanced diet that included, in moderation, stuff usually viewed as "toxic triggers" (coffee, chocolate, fries, and the like), and five were put on a detox regimen. After a week they ran a bunch of tests, including testing for antioxidants and kidney and liver function. The result? No difference. The detoxing didn't do anything.

An interesting analysis done by thirty-six young scientists for an independent organization called the Voice of Young Science (where do I send my check?) looked at the science behind fifteen popular detox products. Among other things, they contacted the manufacturers and asked them for evidence. (Alas, the Clean Cleanse was not studied.) What did they find? *No one* was able to provide any solid evidence to support the detox claims. Remember, they asked the people who made the products! You'd think they'd have a bit of real evidence handy. Also, they found that there wasn't even a consistent or comprehensive definition of *detox*, and, as the study reports, "many of the claims about how the body works were wrong and some were even dangerous." As a result, the thirty-six young scientists concluded: "'Detox' as used in product marketing is a myth."

The reality is that a good study on the efficacy of cleanses would, from a methodological perspective, be fairly complicated, requiring large long-term trials that have individuals on a variety of different cleansing programs and diets. And, ideally, the research method would also elucidate the mechanism of action. So we need to take care not to read too much into experiments such as the one conducted by the BBC. But you simply can't assert, as so many detox sales pitches do, that certain foods magically flush evil toxins out of the system. What toxins? Where do they reside? How do the foods, supplements, vitamins, and so on work?

Many cleansing and detox programs also refer to the idea of creating a healthy gut. Again, this is a big theme for Gwyneth and Dr. Junger. Interesting studies have shown how gut bacteria affect a range of health topics, from psychological well-being to obesity. However, this science, which is still in its early stages, gives cause for caution in the context of cleanses. Before we fiddle with our feces, so to speak, we should recognize that the bacteria that live in our gut play a complex and important role in our health. At the current time, no one (seriously, *no one*) knows if and how we can adjust our diet to alter these microbes in a manner that will maximize health.

"Existing research tells us it is very difficult to reset your [gut bacteria]. You can't easily control what goes on. Even if you can change it, it will just go back to exactly where it was before," Karen Madsen tells me. "Gut bacteria is pretty resilient." Madsen is a professor of gastroenterology at the University of Alberta and codirector of its Centre of Excellence for Gastrointestinal Inflammation and Immunity Research. She is intrigued by my cleansing experiment and suggests that I get my gut material—which is, basically, my feces—tested during and after my cleanse. The process of collecting samples and bringing them to her lab in a (thankfully) opaque plastic container is not fun. But the results are instructive.

Even the idea that we have toxins floating around our bodies is sketchy. Beyond fuzzy references to our dirty environment, the evils of pesticides and pharmaceuticals (for some reason, supplements are OK), rarely do the advocates of cleanses explain what is meant by *toxins*. It is one of those nebulous pseudoscientific terms rolled out by people deliberately avoiding the specificity required for a science-based analysis. It's the modern-day equivalent of "evil spirits," vague enough to mean just about anything while retaining the ring of scientific legitimacy. Every common health complaint—low energy, fatigue, amorphous pain, insomnia, anxiety, general malaise—can be attributed to the existence of toxins. But what, exactly, do the detoxification experts mean? Do they mean the natural poisons that reside in the environment? Do they mean only human-made chemicals? If so, which ones and why? Do they mean junk food? Do they mean all of the above? If so, how are their magical treatments designed to address such vastly different compounds and conditions?

As Joe Schwarcz, director of McGill University's Office for Science and Society, told me when I asked him to sum up the detox fad: "What really needs to be detoxified is the concept of detox."

I CAN'T RESIST commenting on Junger's city-as-a-dirty-fish-tank analogy. The idea that many of us live in toxin-filled, disease-ridden urban bogs is often a core part of the we-must-cleanse narrative. You see it reflected in the images found in Gwyneth's cookbook: Gwyneth sitting in a field in the country. Gwyneth hanging with a friend at a picnic table in the country. Gwyneth riding a red scooter in the country. The whole book has an old-timey country feel. But despite the long-held belief that living in the (allegedly) toxin-free fresh air and wide-open spaces of our rural regions is intrinsically healthy, the available evidence does not support this cliché. While there are certainly health risks associated with both urban and rural settings—and, if you had a time machine, hanging out in pre-sewerage-system London would not be a health-promoting decision—research has consistently shown contemporary cities are healthier than rural retreats, particularly if you are lucky enough to reside in the middle to upper socioeconomic strata (where, I am pretty sure, most "detoxifiers" are found). City dwellers, on average, are slimmer, smoke less, and are more active. Rural dwellers are, on the other hand, more likely to have health issues such as strokes, diabetes, high blood pressure, and some forms of cancer.

A review article published in the *American Journal of Public Health* concluded that "premature mortality (dying before the age of 75) is greater among rural residents than among urban residents." Another article, published in 2014, found that "life expectancy was inversely related to levels of rurality." While much of this difference can be attributed to socioeconomic status, this isn't the whole story. A study published in 2013, for example, found that "youth in rural areas had significantly higher mortality rates than their urban counterparts regardless of deprivation levels [i.e., socioeconomic status]." And other studies have found that the urban poor fare better, from a health perspective, than the non-urban poor. Cities have problems too, of course. There is some evidence that there are higher levels of sexually transmitted disease in urban areas. Also, a 2011 study from Canada found that people living in rural settings had a lower risk of depression, likely because of a stronger sense of community. But contrary to the claims made by many of the detoxification prophets, cities should not be viewed as dirty, disease-causing fish tanks. Indeed, "urbanization appears to be a force for better health," as noted by Christopher Dye, the director of health information at the World Health Organization, in an oft-cited article from the journal *Science*.

Don't get me wrong. I am not a fan of pollution, which cities usually (but not always) have at higher concentrations than in other regions. Pollution is not good for our health. There is even tentative evidence that, for instance, prenatal exposure to a specific pollutant—polycyclic aromatic hydrocarbons, the by-product of burning fossil fuels—can increase the risk of obesity. And I have no objection to the fresh food and active lifestyle so often associated (erroneously, as it turns out) with country life. But there is no evidence that, in the aggregate, cities are inherently unhealthy. There is also no evidence to suggest that living in a city is a reason to cleanse. We urbanites aren't fish in a dirty tank.

SO WHAT WERE the results from my gut test?

The cleanse had absolutely no impact. The Gwyneth cleanse, which is darned extreme, did not change the makeup of the bacteria in my colon. Remember, fixing or "resetting" your gut is one of the alleged goals of cleansing. Madsen's conclusion regarding the condition of my fecal matter is definitive: "Pretty healthy-looking, I would say, and the cleanse did nothing at the phylum level! Your microbes appear to be pretty resilient, which is a good thing."

Inexplicably, I feel a small burst of excreta pride, as if Madsen's assessment of the vast community of microorganisms living in my intestine is a tribute to my character. "Why, thank you . . ."

Stress, Happiness, and Adrenal Fatigue

Many cleanses, including the Clean Cleanse, are also aimed at reducing the emotional and physiological stress caused by a variety of food and environmental toxins. This was a big theme during my discussions with the Clean Program team in Santa Monica. And it is often reported that this is why celebrities go on cleanses: they need to recharge as a result of their hectic celebrity life. Again, this is a point that Gwyneth makes in the preface to *It's All Good*.

So is there any science to suggest this works?

There is some evidence that eating a healthy diet can have a tangible impact on mood. For example, a 2013 study of 281 young adults found that eating fruit and vegetables was associated with a positive emotional state. A similar 2013 study, from Finland, examined the eating habits of more than two thousand individuals and found that a healthy diet, particularly one that emphasizes fruit and vegetables, was protective against depression. Studies have also found that junk food is associated with depression. A 2012 study from Spain followed the eating habits of almost nine thousand individuals and found that "fast-food and commercial baked goods consumption may have a detrimental effect on depression risk." And there is early-stage research showing that the bacteria in our gut can also have an impact on mood. One small study from the University of California at Los Angeles (UCLA), for example, examined the impact on brain function of eating a particular type of yogurt. The study, which included before-and-after brain scans, found that the consumption of probiotic yogurt (which, incidentally, I wasn't allowed to eat while on my cleanse!) altered, for the better, how the brain processes information and reacts to negative stimuli.

There is also research that looks at stress, as measured by such biomarkers as the level of cortisol (often called the stress hormone) in both blood and urine. Studies have found, for example, that a healthy diet may help to reduce stress and protect against its adverse physiological effects. It is also worth noting, however, that this works in the opposite direction too: high stress causes us to eat poorly. A 2013 study from Belgium, for example, measured the cortisol level of 323 children between the ages of five and ten. The measurements were taken three times a day. It was found that higher levels of cortisol (i.e., more stress) were linked to a less-than-healthy diet, including the consumption of fatty foods and more snacks. This may be why we reach for comfort food when stressed out.

While much of the food-and-happiness research is preliminary or marred by methodological limitations (e.g., does eating lots of fruit and vegetables make you happy or do happy people eat lots of fruit and vegetables?), I do believe it is likely that the diet can impact mood and how we handle stress. At a minimum, a healthy diet will make us more resilient and healthier in general, which is, of course, going to help with our emotional well-being.

So, yes, it is possible—in fact, highly probable—that what we put in our mouths can affect our stress level and mood. But there isn't a stitch of evidence to suggest that the particular protocols recommended by the various cleansing programs will have this effect, at least not for the reasons offered by their proponents. Indeed, the preliminary status of this research should remind us that any definitive claim of causation—for example, that certain foods or supplements ease stress and alter hormone levels—is premature. At this stage, the research merely suggests that we should strive to eat a healthy, balanced diet. It does not support the idea that some form of extreme diet—and it is fair to categorize most cleanses as extreme—will improve your long-term emotional well-being and your stress levels as measured by biomarkers.

In fact, at least some research suggests these kinds of diets have the opposite effect, putting our bodies under unnecessary stress. (I certainly felt stressed during my cleanse!) For example, a 2010 study of 121 females found that a diet that greatly restricted calories *increased* blood cortisol levels and the self-reported perception of stress, thereby leading, ironically, to an eventual increase in calorie consumption.

In addition, we need to be cautious in assessing the utility of particular tests as a method for diagnosing an individual's level of stress and well-being. There's little or no evidence to suggest that tests that reveal "sky-high adrenals," for example, have any bearing on health or well-being. While measuring the hormones cortisol and adrenaline—two of the main adrenal hormones—can be useful if there is a demonstrable deficiency or excess (e.g., adrenal insufficiency is a *real* but relatively rare ailment that happens when there's something physically wrong with the adrenal glands), they must be measured throughout the day and at the appropriate time. A 2010 systematic review, which is a rigorous analysis of all the available evidence, looked at the utility of a range of tests, including measurements for cortisol, for the detection of burnout, the term often used to describe the state of stress associated with exhaustion, fatigue, loss of energy, and the like. After carefully analyzing thirty-one studies, the authors concluded: "No potential biomarkers for burnout were found."

Jacques Romney, a University of Alberta colleague and associate professor of endocrinology, agrees with this assessment. He told me that while cortisol and adrenaline are indeed relevant to how the body responds to stress, using a result to determine "how stressed the body might be" is inappropriate. "Cortisol and adrenaline are part of the body's response to stress. However, these hormones naturally fluctuate throughout the day so one cannot pick a certain lab value and determine how stressed one is in day-to-day life."

In fact, the whole concept of "adrenal fatigue" (or "adrenal burnout" or "adrenal exhaustion" or whatever you want to call it) is highly controversial. The theory is that emotional stress and exposure to certain toxins, such as coffee, exhaust the adrenal glands, resulting in a variety of nebulous symptoms (fatigue and feeling overwhelmed, among others). It was partly to relieve my adrenals that I was told to get off coffee as part of my cleanse. As Junger suggests in the book *Clean*, "When caffeine is taken in persistently over a period of time, one can exhaust the adrenal system and not even realize caffeine was the cause."

There is a lot of conflicting (and scientifically inaccurate) information floating around the Internet about this "ailment." Indeed, skeptics have called it an "Internet disease," because, as a commentary in the *Los Angeles Times* noted, adrenal fatigue exists "only in the minds of people who post about [it] on the Internet." It is fair to say that most researchers in the medical and scientific community do not recognize it as a real condition. The endocrinologists I interviewed were blunt in their assessment: adrenal fatigue/exhaustion does not exist, and testing for it is likely useless. A statement from the endocrinologists' professional organization, the Hormone Society, which is the public education arm of the Endocrine Society, is also pretty unequivocal. Specifically, it states: "'Adrenal fatigue' is not a real medical condition. There are no scientific facts to support the theory that long-term mental, emotional, or physical stress drains the adrenal glands and causes many common symptoms." And, just so there is no mistake, they also make the point that "there is no test that can detect adrenal fatigue."

I am not going to take a definitive stand on the concept of adrenal fatigue or the whole idea of testing to see if your "adrenals" are "sky high." I don't need to. My point is more modest: You should not believe anyone who suggests, either explicitly or implicitly, that there is an authoritative biological test for life stress. And you can confidently reject any assertion to the effect that adrenal fatigue/burnout/stress is a well-established condition. More important, given the scientific uncertainty about the nature (or, even, existence) of the problem, don't believe anyone who claims to have a remedy!

Weight Loss

Let's be honest: the primary reason that people cleanse is not for the benefit of some de-stressing, spiritual, soul-centering purification process.

It is for the purpose of weight loss. The main motivation for many of the things we do related to our health, especially dieting, has to do with how we look. And when cleanses are discussed in the popular press, particularly when a celebrity name is invoked, weight loss is almost always the focus. Shape.com, for example, tells us Salma Hayek "credits her slim and sexy shape to the juice cleanses" and that "Beyonce turned to the Master Cleanse Diet to help her drop a reported 20 pounds in less than two weeks." Similarly, Gwyneth's cleanses are often depicted as the secret to her slim body. A February 2014 article in *People* provides a lighthearted analysis of the effectiveness of the cleanses used by Beyoncé, Kyra Sedgwick, Mindy Kaling, and, naturally, Gwyneth. And by effectiveness, *People* means just one thing: weight loss. There is not a single word about actual, scientifically derived evidence in relation to health, but much is said about the number of pounds lost, which ranged from five in twenty-two days to the relatively extreme of twelve in fourteen. So, for all the claims made for them, cleanses are little more than an extreme diet. They are a way to lose weight fast. Indeed, back in Santa Monica, Purohit admitted to me that 80 percent of the company's customers are "interested primarily in weight loss."

How about my cleanse-induced weight loss? Every morning I get naked and anxiously step on our bathroom scale. Gwyneth, Junger, and Purohit will be happy to hear that their cleanse is causing me to lose more than just my dignity. The hard-to-stomach shakes and limited menu options are working their slimming magic. Abracadabra! The weight is disappearing. In my starved state, I can imagine globs of toxins and unhealthy impurities being flushed from my gluten- and coffee-free system.

My morning weigh-in has become the highlight of my day—like when a lab rat gets a hunk of cheese. The inevitable weight loss also serves as a tangible sign that the cleanse is doing something. As I look down at the number on my bathroom scale, I can hear Dr. Junger's soothing voice remind me of how this experience would transform me. Is this what he meant?

But is cleansing a good weight-loss strategy? You can probably guess the answer. I'll start by reviewing what the evidence tells us about weight loss. It isn't pretty. It is, sigh, nearly impossible to keep weight off. Study after study has found that while people can lose weight, sustained weight loss is the true challenge. Even the studies that are structured like clinical trials—that is, the participants are carefully monitored by health-care professionals—have found that the vast majority of people can sustain only modest weight loss, regardless of the type of diet used. (In these studies, successful weight loss is usually defined as keeping off 5 to 10 percent of a person's initial weight—not exactly the beach-ready transformation promised by, to cite one example, the Bikini Detox Diet.) A well-known study published in 2007 carefully analyzed twenty of the most methodologically sound dieting studies to get an idea of how many people actually keep the weight off for two years or longer. They found that the average weight loss was about two pounds and that between one-third and two-thirds of the individuals actually put on more weight than they lost! The authors of the study, led by Traci Mann at the Health and Eating Laboratory at the University of Minnesota, come to the blunt conclusion that dieting simply does not work. Indeed, they suggest that "the most positive conclusion is that dieting slows the slight weight gain that occurs with age among the average non-dieter." Another study of more than nine hundred individuals that was published in the *International Journal of Obesity-Related Metabolism Disorders* found that after fifteen years only 6 percent had managed to keep off just 5 percent of their initial weight, leading the authors to conclude that "long-term weight loss is rare." Is there any reason to think that a cleanse—or, for that matter, any trendy new diet—will, for some magical reason, reverse this trend? No. When you hear about some new approach to dieting, always take a skeptical position. History tells us that the skeptical position will almost always be correct.

You *will* lose weight, temporarily, on a cleanse—as I was clearly doing—but it has absolutely *nothing* to do with the removal of toxins. The weight loss that happens on a cleanse is the direct result of two factors: eating fewer calories, and monitoring what you are eating, which leads to eating fewer calories. OK, it is really the result of one factor: eating fewer calories.

And because many cleanses involve a drastic reduction in calorie intake, the weight often comes off fast. For example, the Master Cleanse—popular with many celebs, including Ashton Kutcher, Ashanti, Pink, and, most famously, Beyoncé in preparation for her role in the movie *Dreamgirls*—is an all-liquid diet based on lemon juice, maple syrup, and cayenne pepper. It involves the consumption of six hundred to seven hundred calories a day, which is much less than half the quantity required by an average woman. It is, quite simply, a crash diet.

Is rapid weight loss a bad idea from the perspective of sustained weight maintenance? Here the data are surprisingly mixed. Intuitively, it seems crazy to put our bodies in starvation mode, slowing the metabolism and, as a result, making it more likely that the weight will come back. Gwyneth herself has made this observation in her well-publicized 2013 critique of the Master Cleanse. (Naturally, she favors Junger's Clean Cleanse, which allows more calories.) But most of the research suggests that, on its own, rapid weight loss isn't particularly harmful, at least in the context of weight loss and *moderate-term* weight management. (You're wrong again, Gwyneth, even when I want you to be right!) A 2013 review of the relevant literature published in the *New England Journal of Medicine* found that rapid weight loss can be just as effective as slow weight loss. A recent study, published in 2013, supports this view. The study compared the weight-loss success of individuals on one-thousand-calorie diets versus those on fifteen-hundred-calorie diets, and the former group fared better, at least after twelve months. (Note: These conclusions do not conflict with the overall weight-loss data. Long-term weight maintenance is *not* the norm. Research has consistently shown that, over time, most dieters struggle to keep weight off.)

Still, there are serious problems with the extreme diet approach. First, as the data I have discussed highlight, it simply isn't going to work for more than a relatively brief period. If sustained weight loss is your goal, the extreme strategy is destined to fail. I contacted Traci Mann, currently a visiting professor at Cambridge University's Institute of Public Health while working on a book that explores the psychology of dieting, to get her view on the idea of cleansing-your-way thin. "The fact is, you can lose weight on pretty much any diet in the short term," she says. "But then the weight comes back on. Given that, why put yourself through the discomfort of a cleanse or any other extreme strategy?" A cleanse is all pain and regain: a lose-lose strategy.

My friend and colleague Dr. Yoni Freedhoff agrees with Mann. He is a weight-loss expert and author of *The Diet Fix*. Freedhoff notes that because cleanses, detoxes, and crash diets often focus on a goal, be it a duration (my twenty-one-day cleanse, for instance), a weight, or an occasion, such as looking good for your *Vogue* cover photo, failure is almost guaranteed. "Many crash dieters revert back to their prediet lifestyles," Freedhoff tells me. "Celebrity diets generally fall into what I would describe as traumatic crash diets. Traumatic in that invariably they involve suffering. Crash in that there's a clear end in sight and usually an abrupt one at that." As noted in the *New England Journal of Medicine* article I quoted earlier, "Obesity is best conceptualized as a chronic condition, requiring on-going management to maintain long-term weight loss." Freedhoff could not agree more. "By considering weight as a chronic condition, and lifestyle changes as its treatment," he tells me, you can never abandon the treatment or "the weight will return." So, if the maintenance of weight loss is your goal, you'd better like your "treatment."

"I've never met anyone who wanted to live on a lemon-pepper cleanse forever," Freedhoff concludes.

If the first problem with cleansing diets is that they don't work, the second problem is that many aren't healthy. They may not, for example, provide adequate nutrients (lemon juice?), and they may erode lean muscle mass. A 2011 study done at the Norwegian Olympic Sport Centre compared the impact of fast and slow weight loss in a group of elite athletes. The researchers found that on all the measured dimensions, including the effect on lean muscle mass, power, and strength, the slow weight loss was superior to the fast weight loss. They recommend that athletes aim for a loss of body weight of about 0.7 percent per week, or about 1.4 pounds if you are a two-hundred-pound man and one pound if you are a 150-pound woman.

Ironically, given that improving how you look is so often a key message attached to the marketing of cleanses, there is also some evidence that cleansing diets may lead to more flab, though the data on this point are inconclusive. At least a few studies have found that repeatedly taking weight off and putting it back on, which is an inevitable consequence of embracing the cleansing approach, is associated with long-term weight gain and the accumulation of abdominal fat. A 2011 study, for example, found that weight cycling, as yo-yo dieting is often called in the academic literature, is associated with a higher-than-average weight and more abdominal fat as compared to non-yo-yo dieters.

I HAVE ABSOLUTELY no idea what Anthony Weiner and Brett Favre were thinking. I cannot imagine what would make a man text a picture of his penis to anyone, especially a woman he is trying to win over. Perhaps it had something to do with celebrity ego and the idea that the famous are exempt from normal rules of behavior—a side effect of the assumption of celebrity authority? But the supposed upside is both delusional and implausible. The practice is all risk, no benefit. In fact, it is my belief that all forms of sexting make absolutely no sense.

But I did it anyway. I couldn't stop myself. I just looked so damn good.

It was the last day of my cleanse. I had made it. It was a wretched grind, but things did get a wee bit better after my caffeine withdrawal subsided. Did I feel pure now? I don't think so. Did I feel happy? Only because it was the last day of my cleanse. Did I feel lighter? Yes, I did.

I lost about nine pounds from my already relatively lean body. Nine pounds in three weeks. Not insignificant. "This is the most toned I'll probably ever be," I mused, as I struck a few muscleman poses for the benefit of no one but my own vain self. And that was when it happened. Without thinking, I grabbed my phone, flexed, snapped a pic in that terrible arm-stretched-out selfie manner, and texted it to my wife.

At least, Mr. Weiner, I kept my pants on. It was just a bit of harmless flexting.

Why So Popular?

Given the sketchy logic and lack of evidence, why are cleanses so popular? I am fascinated by this question, particularly as there are many reputable and easily accessible sources of health information that are unequivocal about the unproven nature of cleanses and detox diets. The Mayo Clinic website, for example, notes that "they're not scientifically proven." And *WebMD*, one of the single most popular sources for health information, notes, "Experts say they are neither necessary nor scientifically proven to work." Yahoo! Health goes even further: "The claims that extreme detoxing will rid your body of toxins, give you more energy and melt away pounds aren't true." But the truth never takes. On the contrary, the popularity of cleanses—and, for that matter, all trendy diets—seems to be growing.

A big part of the story, of course, is that celebrities are vocal supporters of the trend. Celebrities are also under intense pressure to look a certain way. They are both desperate consumers and ardent purveyors of dieting fads. And because they look so darn great, it's easy for the unwary to conclude that cleansing works. But more must be going on. The evidence against the value of cleanses is just so undeniable and the whole concept so silly, it seems unlikely that celebrity endorsements alone would be enough to keep this pseudoscience thriving.

I asked Walter Willett, professor of epidemiology and chair of the Department of Nutrition at the Harvard School of Public Health, to speculate about the continued interest in cleansing despite the clear lack of evidence. His guess: "It is possible that taking a break from the steady overeating that is the norm for most Americans could have some benefit and make people feel better."

I think he is on to something. I do think people view cleanses as a break. But I would take it even further than Willett. I am speculating here, but I think one of the reasons cleanses have so much traction is that they are more than just a break: they are viewed, consciously or unconsciously, as a way to pay for our lifestyle sins. Cleanses are a form of self-flagellation. They are a short-term atonement for bad nutrition choices and consumption excesses. Many celebrities, including Gwyneth, often frame cleanses in these terms, as retribution for holiday indulgences, for example. Gwyneth seems to go on a cleanse every January. ("It is that time of year, folks. I need to lose a few pounds of holiday excess. Anyone else?" she wrote on her Goop website on December 31, 2008.)

Adding to the penance vibe is the reinforcement you get from friends and even strangers. With few exceptions, they offered words of encouragement. I got many in the vein of "Good for you" and "Hang in there." Nobody laughed at me or told me I was nuts. It was generally perceived as a righteous activity, like recycling, driving an electric car, or commuting on a bicycle in the middle of winter. There is also a massive sense of accomplishment when you finish. The mountain summit reached. The marathon completed. So even though the cleanse has no real health benefits, you have a sense that you have done *something*, which likely adds to the placebo effect that leads one to feel pure, happy, and clean.

I've experienced this feeling of triumph over starvation before. When I was fourteen, my older brother, Case, dared me to stop eating. Actually, it was more of a sibling rivalry–fueled contest than a dare. It was summer vacation. We were bored. And Case was reading *Alive*, the book about the soccer team that crashed in the Andes. The survivors were so desperate for food they ate their dead teammates; hence my brother's no-food fixation. Case figured we should give it a try—going without food, that is, not eating human flesh. The rules for our little game were simple: whoever goes the longest without food wins the contest.

I wish I could report that I outlasted my big bro, but, alas, it was a tie. After two full days and much moaning and quarreling, we came to a mutual agreement to stop. (It is hard to imagine a parent of the current hypervigilant variety allowing this to continue beyond morning snack time. It was a different time, as they say.) I vividly remember three things about this tournament. First, I really thought two days without calories was a significant achievement. Second, the first thing I ate when we threw in the towel was an entire row of Chips Ahoy cookies, which I am fairly certain would not be a Gwyneth-approved postcleanse strategy.

And, third—and this is the reason I relate this story—I got a buzz out of the experience.

The popularity of cleansing may be tied to this kind of psychological pick-me-up. It has been noted in some clinical studies that individuals in the first stages of starvation often experience a heightened sense of well-being or bliss. (Note: During my Gwyneth-inspired cleanse, I never felt anything close to euphoria or bliss or even well-being.) For those who experience it, the sensation may be the result of the release of endorphins associated with extreme calorie restriction. Starvation will do that.

Of course, the other reason they are so popular is that they lead to short-term weight loss. I lost weight. Again, starvation will do that.

The No-Gimmick Cleanse

Perhaps I should simply stop fighting it: people want a cleanse. If you can't beat them, join them, as they say. So here is the Caulfield Cleanse. It is simple. It is cheap. In fact, it might save you money. You don't need to buy any useless supplements, vitamins, or special juices. You don't need to consume fancy powder drinks or avoid gluten, coffee, or even (moderate) amounts of alcohol. And I guarantee it will work.

Step 1: Cleanse your system of all the pseudoscientific babble that flows from many celebrities, celebrity physicians, and the diet industry.

Step 2: Supplement with a daily dose of healthy skepticism.

Step 3: Detoxify your system with evidence produced by the scientific community and disseminated by independent entities (a favorite source: Cochrane Collaboration, a nonprofit entity that prepares rigorous systematic reviews).

Step 4: Watch your calorie intake (diet diaries are a terrific and evidence-based strategy), and eat lots of fruits and vegetables (aim for about 50 percent of what goes in your mouth).

I am only half joking. Virtually every science-informed expert I contacted said the same thing. People should forget about cleanses and trendy diets and concentrate on consuming an appropriate amount of calories (for most, this is between eighteen hundred and twenty-two hundred per day) and eating in a nutritious manner, which means fruits, vegetables, whole grains, nuts, legumes, lean protein (including fish), and a bit of dairy. In fact, the preceding sentence captures almost all you need to know about a healthy diet. You can ignore everything else.

While there is more to a healthy diet than just fruits and vegetables, this is a logical place to start. If we could just increase the percentage of people who eat an adequate amount of fruits and vegetables, we could have a real, long-term impact on the health of the population. Few of us eat enough. Research from the United States says that, in 2009, fewer than 14 percent ate the recommended amount. A 2013 study from Sweden involving more than seventy thousand people, for example, found that eating fruits and vegetables was associated with a longer and healthier life. Another massive study, also from 2013, followed almost half a million people and found a similar reduction of mortality, particularly in the context of cardiovascular disease. Other recent research has found that fruits and vegetables may protect against mental health issues and assist with sustained weight maintenance. Also, making this conscious effort to consume more fruits and veggies may allow people to feel like they are committing to a fresh start or "resetting" their system, two concepts that seem central to the popularity of the cleansing strategy.

So keep it simple. Ignore the hype. Remember, history tells us all dieting trends are likely to be wrong. They never work. What follows are just a few examples of topics and trends that are distorted by celebrity culture's spin.

Coffee: "Today I quit my beloved coffee & make the switch to vitamin B complex," Katy Perry told the world via Twitter. Why would anyone quit coffee for health reasons? Coffee is *good* for you. There is no evidence that coffee exhausts your adrenals or is taxing your detox organs (sigh), as the cleansing gurus of the world would have us believe. And there is lots of evidence that it protects against a variety of ailments, including Parkinson's, type 2 diabetes, and liver cancer. It also improves brain function and athletic performance. Drink up, Ms. Perry. Coffee is making you healthier. (Full disclosure: my deep love of coffee may influence my interpretation of the data, despite my halfhearted effort to remain semi-objective about this matter.)

Vitamins and supplements: What about Perry's much-publicized decision to start consuming a boatload of vitamins? In May 2013, for example, she tweeted a picture of herself to her then–46 million followers; it showed her holding up three massive bags of pills, which, apparently, she gulps down upon rising, with breakfast and at dinner. "I'm all about that supplement & vitamin LYFE!" she said.

In fact, most studies suggest that taking vitamins and supplements—which I was required to do as part of my cleanse—is usually completely unnecessary and might even be harmful. A study of almost forty thousand women, for instance, found no benefit to taking a range of supplements and concluded that there was "little justification for the general and widespread use of dietary supplements." Research has also found that vitamin C does not prevent cancer or, for that matter, colds; supplementation with some vitamins (e.g., A and E) may increase the risk of certain cancers; taking supplements with omega-3 may increase the risk of prostate cancer; and, according to a report from the Harvard School of Public Health, further supplementation with high doses of the vitamin Bs "has not been found to be beneficial and might actually cause harm."

Other studies have found that many supplements are often not what they say they are. Indeed, chances are Perry has no idea what she is gobbling in her attempt to live a healthier LYFE. A 2013 study from the University of Guelph, for example, did a blind study of commercially available supplements and found that "most of the herbal products were of poor quality, including considerable product substitution, contamination and use of fillers." Remarkably, these researchers found some product substitution—the use of another, unlabeled herb in the place of the main ingredient—in products of 83 percent of the companies tested. In other words, only 17 percent of the companies were providing products that matched what the label said. This is, of course, both dangerous and unethical. It should not be forgotten that the massive supplement and vitamin industry, worth, by some estimates, approximately $60 billion worldwide, is about profits and moving product. Because of the bucks to be made, many pharmaceutical companies have recently acquired companies that produce supplements. Since it is not a tightly regulated industry, this situation should surprise no one.

You should strive to get all your vitamins from the food you eat, not from pills. Even in the context of vitamin D, a supplement that has received a lot of attention in the popular press, the evidence is more equivocal than often portrayed. A 2010 report from the US Institute of Medicine (IOM) of the National Academies of Science found that while vitamin D plays a key role in bone health, most of us get enough from food and sun. It reported that current evidence "does not support other benefits of vitamin D" intake and that the higher levels associated with supplement intake may be harmful. So more is not better. A more recent analysis, published in 2013 by the US Preventive Services Task Force, found that even in the context of bone health, there is still insufficient evidence about the benefits to recommend use of vitamin D supplements for most populations. A subsequent study, published in late 2013 in the journal the *Lancet*, has taken it even further, finding that vitamin D is not necessary for bone health in otherwise healthy individuals. And yet another study, this one from 2014 and published in the *Lancet Diabetes & Endocrinology*, concluded that vitamin D had little effect on a range of health problems, including cardiovascular disease, mood disorders, and weight gain. The *New York Times* quoted the lead author of the study as saying, "Unfortunately, there is probably no benefit to expect from vitamin D supplementation in normally healthy people."

I am not saying that there is never a reason to take a supplement. Pregnant women, for example, have particular needs, and some individuals may have clear, clinically determined deficiencies. And data on some supplements, such as vitamin D, are still being compiled. But, to date, there is absolutely no evidence that living a "supplement & vitamin LYFE" is a good idea. Most of the relevant science suggests the opposite.

Colon cleanses: The idea that a colon cleanse removes toxins and promotes health is so ridiculous that it is a pretty good test for quacks. If a book, health-care practitioner, TV doctor, magazine columnist, or blogger recommends a colon cleanse, also known as a colonic or colonic hydrotherapy, you can flush all their advice down the toilet.

On this subject, I don't need to mince words. Colon cleanses don't work and are potentially harmful. Even though celebs like Madonna, Leonardo DiCaprio, and Britney Spears may have embraced the fecal flush, the whole concept is nonsense. As noted in a 2011 review of the relevant scientific literature, there are "no scientifically robust studies in support of this practice." Other reviews have come to a similar conclusion. Not only does it do no good, the practice also is likely to be harmful. It can result in nausea, vomiting, infection, and, in rare circumstances, the perforation of the bowel. It can also adversely impact your electrolytes and your gut's natural bacteria. All these potential risks are, of course, increased the more frequently you do colon cleanses.

Incidentally, in his book *Clean*, Junger recommends colonic hydrotherapy—which is, as he explains, "the injection of pure water delivered at low pressure into the colon and then drawn out." He further advises thus: "You can have as many [colonic] treatments during Clean as you like, depending on your budget and schedule. (I've even had patients who got them daily during their detox.)" I'll leave it to you to determine the degree to which the recommendation of daily colon cleanses impacts his credibility.

While I followed all the rules associated with my Clean Cleanse, I could not bring myself to implement this part of the program. Unnecessary. Unsafe. Unscientific. And kind of disgusting.

Juicing: Forbes recently called juicing a "celebrity trend gone wild." Which, given the huge increase in the sale of both premade juices and home juicing machines, is a more than fair assessment. If you do a Google Images search for "celebrity juicing," you get pictures of Hilary Duff,

Jennifer Garner, Nicole Richie, Orlando Bloom, Blake Lively, Olivia Wilde, and, of course, Gwyneth holding some kind of (usually green) juice concoction.

The premise behind juicing is that removing the harder-to-digest fiber (many of the trending juices are "pressed") concentrates the vitamins and makes them easier to digest. The problem is that, once again, there is no evidence to support the concept that juicing is a better way to get our fruits and vegetables, lose weight, remove toxins, or ingest calories. I also could not find a cogent explanation for why we need to absorb our vitamins quickly—presuming, of course, that juicing allows this to happen—or give our digestive tract a break from fiber. Indeed, studies have found that drinking your calories is far from ideal because liquids don't make humans feel as full as solid foods do. Think about how you feel after eating an actual apple, banana, and half a cup of blueberries and compare that to how you feel after drinking juice with the same ingredients. Not the same. A study from 2013 concluded that people find solid meals more satisfying than liquids—even meal-replacement shakes. (No surprise here, given my experience with the less than gratifying Clean Cleanse shakes.) Other studies have shown that the consumption of liquid instead of solid calories is associated with increased calorie intake and a higher body mass index (BMI).

A 2013 investigation by the Harvard School of Public Health confirmed the tremendous benefits of eating an adequate amount of fruits and vegetables but, once again, found juice to be problematic. The research looked at data from almost 190,000 participants and found that individuals who ate whole fruits—especially blueberries, grapes, and apples—reduced their risk for type 2 diabetes by 23 percent. But individuals who drank one or two servings of fruit juice actually *increased* their risk. So put down that expensive, trendy, kale-infused liquid and pick up a real apple.

OK, to be fair, there is nothing inherently dangerous about juicing or the closely related smoothie, unlike colonics. (Smoothies probably are slightly better for you, because they are usually made by blending the entire fruit and, as a result, include more fiber—but the juicing/smoothie jargon is a bit slippery.) And, I suppose, juicing can be a way to get a more varied intake of fruits and vegetables. But there is nothing magically healthy about juicing or juice products. Unless some medical reason keeps you from masticating—perhaps a paparazzo's camera broke your jaw—juicing shouldn't be a nutrition strategy. This fad is based on such a thin rationale that it may fade soon. Indeed, the whole juicing scene is getting pretty wacky. "All our juices are handcrafted—it's more of an art," one New York juicing company owner told the *New York Daily News.* When people start talking about handcrafted juice, we are nearing the point where Fonzie is warming up the speedboat in preparation for his jump over a cold-pressed, organic juice–filled shark tank.

Organic: This one is tough. I need to tread carefully or the hate mail will flow. It is a complex topic, and many feel passionate about eating organic. As usual, of course, celebs lead the way. "I find the most satisfying food is food that's full of life, so it's raw and clean and organic," says the model Miranda Kerr. And, naturally, Gwyneth and Dr. Junger are big on organic. The word *organic* appears often on the pages of *The Clean Cleanse* manual (actual count: twelve mentions in a forty-eight-page document).

But despite the deep attachment that many individuals and organizations have to organic food, the evidence about its benefits is far from conclusive. The best available research suggests that organic food—which, by the way, can be tough to define—is not nutritionally superior to conventionally grown products. Given that studies report that personal health is a key reason that people buy organic, and given the enthusiasm with which the advocates of organic food endorse the practice, it is important to note that this is the conclusion formed by numerous, respected organizations and researchers. For example, a 2009 study by a group from Public Health and Policy, London School of Hygiene and Tropical Medicine, did a meta-analysis of the scientific evidence and found "no evidence of a difference in nutrient quality between organically and conventionally produced foodstuffs." A more recent study, published in 2012 by a team from Stanford University, agreed, noting that there is no strong evidence that "organic foods are significantly more nutritious than conventional foods."

Some studies have found that some organic foods have slightly more micronutrients and less pesticide residue, but despite these findings, no good studies "have directly demonstrated health benefits or disease protection as a result of consuming an organic diet," according to a review published in the journal *Pediatrics* in 2012. In other words, even if there are small differences, there is no evidence to suggest these differences are clinically relevant. Indeed, most of the available data suggest they are not—but, to be fair, more research on this point would be helpful. (The micronutrient concern seems a bit ridiculous. The differences, if there are any, are so small that a tiny additional bite of a conventionally grown item would more than compensate.) Consumers also should recognize that organic farming also uses pesticides, though only "natural" ones. But this doesn't mean they are necessarily healthier or better for the environment. Steven Novella reports in *Science-Based Medicine*: "There is little to no evidence that these organic pesticides are less harmful for consumers or the environment. It is just assumed that they are based upon the naturalistic fallacy." While not all will agree with this opinion (I do!), it is important to recognize the scientific uncertainty about the supposed benefits of organic food. Here is just one example that highlights the uncertainty: a University of Guelph study from 2010 found "organic approved insecticides had a similar or even greater negative impact on several natural enemy species in lab studies, were more detrimental to biological control organisms in field experiments, and had higher [environmental impact] at field use rates."

A recent analysis by the Canadian government found that almost 50 percent of organic food has residue from synthetic pesticides. One official with the Organic Trade Association told CBC News that this level of contamination likely indicates deliberate use of synthetic pesticides by some organic farmers.

Despite what the science tells us, people will, no doubt, continue to purchase organic products. Buying organic food is, like many purchasing choices, as much a way of expressing a worldview—or even a form of self-expression—as it is a diet choice. People buy organic for many reasons, including taste, concern about the environment, and a desire to help the local economy. For some, it is also associated with a desire to represent a particular alternative, anticorporate lifestyle. There are two ironic twists to this personal-branding side of organic food. First, organic food is now a multibillion-dollar industry that preys on and profits from the consumer's desire to project a particular healthy and environmentally friendly ethos. Big Food companies like Kellogg and PepsiCo now own many organic food brands. As noted in a 2012 *New York Times* article by Stephanie Strom that outlined the corporatization of organic food (or, as the author calls it, Big Organic): "Pure, locally produced ingredients from small family farms? Not so much anymore." Second, an interesting and, to be honest, kind of funny study explored the degree to which purchasing organic food influenced moral attitudes and altruistic behavior. Given the degree to which organic food is marketed with moral overtones—organic brands have names such as Honest Team, Purity Life, Seeds of Change, Living Tree Community—the author was curious about whether organic food affected how people behaved. The study came to the paradoxical conclusion that being exposed to organic food does not make individuals into caring, open-minded hippies. It makes people more self-righteous, judgmental, and *less* altruistic. This admittedly small study led an editor at the *Atlantic* to write this headline: "Does Organic Food Make You a Judgmental Jerk?" For me, it highlights the complex relationship between food and our beliefs. What we eat reflects, and perhaps shapes, how we see the world.

If you enjoy the taste of organic food (although numerous studies have found little evidence to support the "tastes better" claim, including a 2012 study that found blindfolded consumers actually preferred the taste of *conventionally* grown tomatoes!) or like the idea of buying your food at a farmers' market, then, by all means, carry on. (Hey, I do it too.) But do not believe any of the rhetoric that suggests you'll reap any health benefits. Don't believe the claims that conventional foods contain fatigue-generating toxins or that they will exhaust your adrenals. There is absolutely no good evidence to show that this is true.

Gluten: Near the beginning of the movie *This Is the End*, Seth Rogen, playing himself, tells his buddy Jay Baruchel that he is on a cleanse and that we should all stop eating gluten. "Whenever you feel shitty, that's because of gluten," Rogen explains. "*Gluten* is a vague term. It's something that's used to categorize things that are bad. Ya know? Calories, that's a gluten. Fat, that's a gluten." It is a hilarious scene. And it is spot on. The bit captures the current insanity surrounding gluten and, more broadly, wheat, which have become the new food devils. Every conceivable human health problem has been attributed to the consumption of gluten and/or wheat, including fatigue, obesity, diabetes, migraines, Alzheimer's, and even autism. (This last one has been pushed by, no surprise here, Jenny McCarthy.)

The demonization of gluten, which is a protein found in wheat and other grains, can be traced to best-selling books such as *Wheat Belly* and, naturally, advocacy by hordes of gluten-free celebrities, including Gwyneth and basketball star Steve Nash. Gluten-free foods have become a massive industry. Some estimates put the size of the gluten-free food market at about $6 billion, as approximately 20 percent of the US population now buys gluten-free products, and as many as a third say they would like to cut down on gluten. The primary reasons for the popularity of this diet approach are, first, the belief that it is healthier and, second, that it will lead to weight loss. Indeed, a survey of more than two hundred dietitians pegged gluten free as the most popular diet and weight-loss approach of 2013.

But what does the relevant science say?

Unfortunately, the evidence does not provide straightforward answers. Let me start with the facts that seem pretty certain. Despite claims to the contrary, no credible study has shown that gluten/wheat is the cause of the current obesity epidemic. There is also no credible evidence to suggest that eliminating gluten and wheat from your diet is a wise lifestyle choice—unless, of course, you have a clinically identified reason for doing so (for example, if you are one of the approximately 1 in 141 who have celiac disease). Nor is it a proven weight-loss strategy. In fact, some studies have found that eliminating gluten can lead to weight gain. A 2006 study, for example, followed 371 gluten-free dieters—these were individuals with celiac disease—and found that 82 percent had gained weight after two years. Not so surprising, perhaps, given that there is no reason to assume gluten-free food has fewer calories. One review article nicely summarized the research on this point: "It is important to note that gluten-free does not necessarily mean low-energy [i.e., low-calorie], and some gluten-free products actually have a greater energy value than corresponding gluten-containing foods."

There are many anecdotal reports of gluten-free weight-loss success, often connected to some superslim celeb. For example, a 2013 article in the *Daily Mail* headlined "Gluten-Free Devotee Miley Cyrus Shows Off Her Flat Stomach" reports that the "bread, pasta and pizza-free way of life seems to be paying off for Miley Cyrus."

Ignore this kind of hype. Anecdotes and personal testimonials—no matter how compelling and belly-button revealing—are not good science. The evidence shows that whole grains are actually good for us. They are, among other things, full of fiber and vitamins. Studies have consistently found that the healthiest diets, such as the Mediterranean diet, contain whole grains.

It seems likely that much of the gluten-free craze is the result of celebrity culture and opportunistic marketing. Gluten-free products are generally expensive and, one can assume, highly profitable. A recent editorial in the *British Medical Journal* goes so far as to suggest that the entire area is "being driven by profit and market forces, not medical forces." As a 2011 consumer information document published by the US Food and Drug Administration put it: "For people not sensitive to gluten, there is no health benefit to a gluten-free diet."

OK, so going gluten free isn't a smart weight-loss or nutrition strategy, but what about the ever-increasing number of people who report sensitivity to gluten? I want to emphasize, again, that I am not referring to individuals who have celiac disease, which is a condition that can be diagnosed through laboratory tests. For people with this relatively rare condition, avoiding gluten is necessary. Here, I am referring to individuals who do not have celiac disease but still feel that gluten is causing symptoms such as stomach pain, diarrhea, bloating, and fatigue. This is where things get a bit confusing.

On one side of the argument is the dubious nature of the evidence. For example, there are no definitive biomarkers (e.g., blood tests, tissue samples) that are associated with gluten sensitivity, and the best studies have failed to clearly identify the condition. This has led many researchers to question the very existence of nonceliac gluten sensitivity. A recent study from Australia, for example, used a sophisticated double-blind approach (i.e., neither the researchers nor the research participants knew whether the food was truly gluten free) and found no evidence of gluten sensitivity. An editorial accompanying the study, which was published in the journal *Gastroenterology*, suggests the "study calls into question the very existence of NCGS [nonceliac gluten sensitivity] as a discrete entity."

I contacted two of the study's authors, Jessica Biesiekierski and Peter Gibson, of the Department of Gastroenterology at Monash University in Australia. Both have been researching this issue for years. The results, as Gibson told me, were pretty definitive. "Our recent study using the 'gold standard' of repeated double-blinded placebo-controlled re-challenge showed, in a population of patients who believed they were gluten sensitive, that none really were." To repeat, *none* of them were. Naturally, even a definitive finding like this does little to convert believers. You can sense Gibson's frustration. "The take [on this study] by some was that we picked the wrong patients and that we got it wrong in some way. In other words, pseudoscience is more reliable than real science."

Biesiekierski agrees with Gibson but concedes that the growth in self-reported sensitivity hints that something may be going on. "I think there is *some* evidence that NCGS *may* exist, but probably only in a *very small number* of people. However, I am still skeptical and ultimately the existence of NCGS will remain unsubstantiated until there is more definitive, reproducible research."

Some medical researchers have speculated that people feel better when they go gluten free simply because they start eating better (e.g., more fruit and vegetables)—and less. On the other side of the argument are the studies that have tried to map the incidence of gluten sensitivity. Dr. Alessio Fasano from the Center for Celiac Research at Massachusetts General Hospital in Boston, for example, using both self-report and clinical investigations, has suggested that as much as 6 percent of the population could have some degree of sensitivity. A more recent study from Columbia University put that incidence at a much lower 0.55 percent. But neither conclusion appears to be definitive, and the academic debate about the nature and incidence of gluten sensitivity seems likely to rage for years to come. The bottom line: the science on nonceliac gluten sensitivity is still emerging. As another review of the relevant research, published in September 2013, put it: "Non-celiac gluten sensitivity is an entity awaiting validation, better diagnostic criteria, and, if it does exist, pathogenic mechanisms."

So Seth Rogen was right: *gluten* is a pretty vague term. Still the bulk of the science tells us that most of us do not need to shy away from gluten or wheat. Whatever Gwyneth and Miley may tell you, the science doesn't agree.

Three Weeks After My Cleanse

All the weight is back on my old, flabby frame. Infuriating. No more flexting. Phone stays in pocket.

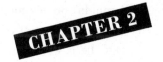

CHAPTER 2

Beauty Tips from Beautiful People

"Your facial routine is pretty time consuming," my wife, Joanne, says to me as I carefully apply my moisturizing sunscreen, the last phase of my morning skin-care and antiaging program. It is early, she needs to get to work, and she obviously doesn't appreciate my meticulous rinsing procedure. Chop, chop! Let's get a move on!

Until recently, my approach to skin care had been exceedingly time efficient. It included precisely nothing. Zip. I washed my face with plain, cheap, bulk-purchased soap, which I used only when something on my face needed washing. I didn't even use shaving cream. I just dragged a crappy disposable razor over some of that plain soap. I rarely wore a hat when outside (bad) and almost never put on sunscreen (very bad). But I am a changed man. Twice daily my old skin is now pampered like the Stanley Cup—game seven, third period.

Not long ago I flew to Calgary to meet with an old friend and re-spected dermatologist, Kirk Barber, who is now a professor in the Faculty of Medicine at the University of Calgary. I met Barber when I was an undergrad, nearly thirty years ago, and consequently he has seen me at my sartorial worst. I believe the day of our first encounter I sported a faux hawk, a dangly lightning-bolt earring, and a too-tight biker jacket. All things considered, I figured I couldn't do anything to further humiliate myself in his eyes. This makes him the perfect confidant for my latest vanity project. More important, he is well positioned to help me sift through all the myths and truths about skin-care and antiaging practices.

I told Barber that I wanted to adopt a typical skin-care routine, something that an aging celebrity might use on a daily basis. My goal was both to experience a comprehensive skin-care regime (something I hadn't attempted since I stressed about acne in high school) and to determine whether, in fact, a high-tech routine can make a difference. Are beauty products worth it? Since I was interested in experiencing what people actually do to protect and enhance their skin—and not, necessarily, what the evidence says we should be doing—Barber introduced me to Marie, who ran a "skin science" clinic next to his office. This was not a medical office but a clinic that provides cosmetic services and products aimed at helping people enhance the look and condition of their skin. "I am, really, a skin coach," Marie told me as she showed me around the office. She has a graduate degree in microbiology, is infectiously good-natured, and has absolutely flawless skin.

Marie invited me into her all-white office: white table, white walls, white chairs, and white machinery. I told her about my project and hinted that I was pretty skeptical about the whole skin-care industry. She ignored the implied criticism and launched into a heartfelt lecture on the benefits of various products and skin-care routines. She also had a great deal to say about the condition of my skin. Not good. Using a machine that would be at home on the bridge of the starship *Enterprise*—the new, J. J. Abrams–directed *Enterprise*, not the old cardboardy-looking ship from TV—she took a picture of my face that, she explained, would provide a host of information about the treatment she would recommend.

The machine produces a series of colorful, and less-than-flattering, images of my face, each highlighting a particular skin property, such as wrinkles, redness, sun damage, and pore quality. Now, this machine looked impressive but despite a good bit of digging I could not find an independent analysis of its clinical value. The website for the company that manufactures the machine states, among other things, that the company has "deployed [their] complexion analysis software as a sales tool to promote" brands of cosmetic products, that it "impressively increases business in all of your skin care services," and that the machine "was never intended for clinical trials." Reading between the lines (or, actually, simply reading the lines), it seems the company views this machine as a way to move product. So there are reasons to be dubious about the meaning and relevance of the results. Still, the premise of the device, taking pictures of my face to assess its condition, is not farfetched. I go with the flow.

The good news: my wrinkle situation is great. For my age and ethnicity, I have fewer wrinkles than about 95 percent of the population. It must be all that plain, bulk-purchased soap. The bad news: my pore situation is catastrophic. The picture reveals that I have more than one thousand clogged pores on my face. "You have the worst pores I have seen in over eight years," Marie tells me with a shake of her head. I stifle the sudden impulse to dash out of the room to scrub my filthy face with an industrial-strength solvent.

To be honest, I have never noticed, and no one has ever commented on, my poor-pore predicament. My wife has never mentioned it. Nor have my singularly candid children and brothers ever mocked me about it. Nevertheless, according to the picture produced by Marie's *Star Trek* machine, this was a serious cosmetic problem that needed fixing. I left Marie's office with a bag full of high-end beauty products, including a cleansing-exfoliation gel that was designed to decongest aging skin, another cleaning lotion to control bacteria, a nighttime moisturizer that claims to be specifically designed for bad pores, and a morning moisturizer that doubles as a sunblock. The plan was to use these products morning and night for three months.

Big Beauty and the Evidence Challenge

The beauty industry is, of course, massive. It involves everything from teeth-whitening toothpaste to ridiculously expensive shampoo that will transform your hair "from ordinary to extraordinary," if you believe an advertisement for a product that contains white truffles and caviar and costs more than $60 for an 8.5-ounce bottle. It involves celebrity-endorsed cosmetics, perfumes, and a host of fashion products. And it involves numerous fitness and slimming gimmicks. I will make no attempt to undertake a comprehensive analysis of every allegedly beautifying product that is touched by a celebrity. The number is infinite. It's enough to know that the beauty industry is a huge cultural force in a tight, symbiotic relationship with celebrities and the celebrity-oriented media. The size and influence of this industry creates challenges for anyone seeking to get to the truth about the products it makes and promotes.

In my research I worked hard to find experts who could provide a reasonably independent view of the alleged benefits of the myriad beauty and antiaging products and services. This proved to be much more difficult than I anticipated. Many experts I contacted were not independent scientists but dermatologists who also had a clinical practice and, as such, benefit (some greatly) from a thriving industry. I am *not* saying that physicians knowingly twist information about the efficacy of beauty treatments, but there is ample evidence that such conflicts of interest can have an impact on how research is presented and interpreted.

In addition, little literature produced by independent researchers is out there. For many beauty products, there seem to be either no data or only small studies produced by the proponents of the product. To some degree, this is understandable. Government research entities, such as the US National Institutes of Health or the Canadian Institutes of Health Research, have little interest in funding big double-blind placebo-controlled trials on the efficacy, for instance, of bird-poop facial cream. So there isn't a lot of good science to draw on. To make matters worse, the popular press is rarely critical of new beauty products. While I found many excellent and balanced media stories on beauty treatments (usually panning them), the vast majority of articles simply trumpet their alleged value, using vague descriptors such as *revitalize* and *radiate*. Rarely did I find any real evidence or any expertise beyond personal testimonies (which I don't need to remind you are not evidence). The so-called experts who are quoted in these articles are often part of the beauty industry or individuals with no research background. To cite just one example, a frequently quoted "expert" who is a beauty columnist for a well-known women's health magazine, and an advocate for all things pseudoscientific, describes herself as an eco-advisor, television personality, and restaurateur—interesting resume, for sure, but hardly a background that lends itself to a critical analysis of beauty products. And, remember, publishers don't generally sell magazines by reminding readers that nothing works. And they're unlikely to make a practice of denigrating the industry that purchases so much of their advertising space. So they have a built-in tendency to recommend beauty products by either explicitly or implicitly suggesting that they work.

Consequently, getting straight answers about antiaging and beauty products is nearly impossible. There exists a confluence of fact-twisting forces: lots of money to be made by manufacturers and providers, huge advertising campaigns that deploy vast quantities of pseudoscientific gobbledygook, a lack of independent research and information, and consumers who desperately want the products to do for them what is claimed. The cumulative impact of all these forces results in a massive bias toward representing a product or procedure as effective. I call this the "beauty industry efficacy bias," or BIEB for short. Sadly, few social forces are on the other side of the BIEB equation, so the BIEB reigns supreme. (Note: The link between the BIEB acronym and Justine Bieber's nickname was not intentional—honest!—but it does work well. This struggling singer occupies a hefty hunk of the celebrity-culture space and has endorsed a variety of beauty products.)

Given the existence of the BIEB, we should always bring a furiously critical eye to the assessment of any claim made by Big Beauty. Phrases such as "clinically proven" or "dermatologist approved" have little meaning because they could refer to almost anything. For example, what kind of study led to the representation that a given product was clinically proven? Did the manufacturers simply ask a couple of buyers? Do not be fooled by this kind of language, particularly when the presence of the BIEB makes critical analysis of the claims unlikely.

In addition to the BIEB dilemma, history tells us that a skeptical position is almost always correct. As with trendy diets, after the passage of a bit of time it almost invariably becomes clear that the alleged benefits associated with some new, exciting antiaging beauty product can't live up to the hype.

Celebrity Skin, Celebrity Solutions

"I'll have the omelet," I tell the waiter.

"Excellent choice," he replies.

I'm sitting on the porch of a Beverly Hills restaurant called The Ivy with the singular purpose of looking for celebrity skin. Facial skin, that is. I am in the Hollywood area, I'm researching celebrity dermatological routines, and I figure I might as well get a look at the real deal. I want to compare my normal-person epidermis to the unique and otherworldly qualities of a face that has been properly pampered. Do celebrities really radiate? Do they glow? I figure that The Ivy is my best bet because it is a well-known hangout for celebs. As one Los Angeles travel website notes, "The attention-hungry frequently sit on the front patio, where only a white picket fence separates them from prying lenses." That is exactly where I am sitting, and, as luck would have it, the prying lenses are about eight feet away.

Sitting at a table in front of me is a group of beautiful young women. They are attracting a gaggle of photographers so, I am guessing, one or more of the women must be reasonably famous. While I like to believe that I am in touch with popular culture, I have absolutely no idea who they are. One looks vaguely familiar—perhaps she's a model?—but I can't place her. I desperately want to snap a picture for future research, but the waiter has told me to put away both my phone and computer. (For some reason, the producer-sounding guy sitting nearby is allowed to keep his electronics in plain view. Do I have a stalker vibe?) I manage to sneak a picture of my outrageously delicious omelet—which was only slightly less expensive than a slab of plutonium—but no picture of customers opposite. These women, who look young enough to be in high school, do indeed have categorically impeccable skin. Flawless. I might even detect a slight glow.

Just as I get perilously close to a staring intensity that I fear will attract we-must-ask-you-to-leave attention, one of the women starts primping. She is fussing with her hair, applying stuff to her lips, and going through other such rituals. She then pops up from her chair and starts posing for the paparazzi. Hand on hip. Hair fling. Over the shoulder. Big smile. Sexy smile. Pouty face. The cameras snap obediently in response. This goes on for about a minute, and then a waiter dolefully shoos the photographers away. The young woman plops back into her seat and continues chatting with her friends as if nothing has happened. It almost seemed staged. Perhaps it was.

I realize this is an utterly silly experiment. Of course, twentysomething model-type women, and probably most of humanity, have skin superior to my blotchy, clogged Celtic hide. I didn't really expect to find any dermatologically challenged celebrities. But the incident perfectly frames the role of celebrity culture in the realm of beauty. The beauty standard set by celebrity culture and the beauty industry is often calibrated by just the kind of photographer-celebrity interaction I witnessed while inhaling an overpriced brunch. Young women posing for pictures.

IN MANY WAYS, celebrity culture sits at the center of the massive skin-care and antiaging industry. Some estimates put the global skin-care market at approximately $80 billion, and it has been suggested that the entire antiaging industry will be worth almost $300 billion by 2015. Celebrity culture helps to set the benchmark for how our skin is supposed to look. (In a word: young—as nicely illustrated by my neighbors at The Ivy.) Celebrities are increasingly used to market skin-care products. And through their well-publicized beauty rituals they help to perpetuate an assortment of antiaging and skin-care beliefs—the vast majority of which are unscientific and completely unproven.

Celebrities are at once the victims and generators of beauty myths. They primp for paparazzi, thus helping to create the standard by which we all are measured. But, having set the standard, they must also strive to maintain it. People in the entertainment industry, especially women, are under unbelievable pressure to appear young. I heard this message repeatedly from directors and actors and from the dermatologists who work with them. This being the case, we should, I suppose, cut celebrities a bungee-cord length of slack when it comes to their choice of beauty regimens. Desperation can obscure rational reflection and prompt experimentation with anything that might help to maintain a "youthful glow."

But the beauty-regimen quackery is hard to take when the pseudoscientific mumbo jumbo is peddled to the masses through interviews, endorsements, and celebrity gossip. The popular press usually presents this stuff without a scintilla of critical analysis. On the contrary. At times there is a mocking tone—it is tough to report on David and Victoria Beckham's use of bird-poo facials without at least a hint of tongue-in-cheek-ness— but more often than not, the beauty products are presented as new, exciting, and effective. This is the BIEB at work.

A cursory scan of popular newspapers and magazines turns up an overwhelming number of questionable celebrity beauty tips. Virtually every magazine with a focus on fashion, celebrities, health, or fitness offers regular advice on skin care and combating aging. Most newspapers have a weekly style or beauty section. At any given moment, probably hundreds of beauty-related recommendations are sitting on the average midsize magazine stand. And all these stories are almost completely devoid of any reference to credible evidence. Beauty advice is a science-free zone. Anything goes.

It is no surprise, then, that celebrity antiaging activities, whether mildly nutty or utterly senseless, usually evade informed scrutiny. For example, many newspapers and magazines reported, most without a single reference to science, that Kate Middleton used a bee-venom facial as a needle-free shortcut to youthful, line-free skin. (Isn't the princess *already*, chronologically speaking, pretty darn youthful?) I read numerous stories about celebrities using placental face masks, which were described as coming from some ultrapure sheep in the mountains of New Zealand. Not one of these stories questioned the effectiveness of sheep afterbirth as an antiaging ointment, and several said it worked. A similarly uncritical attitude characterized stories about Demi Moore's famous leech therapy (which, as one source states, "cleanses the blood, improves circulation and boosts tissue healing") and the use of snails on the face, favored by celebs such as Katie Holmes, that, as reported by *Glamour*, leave a trail of "mucus that's packed with proteins, antioxidants, and hyaluronic acid, which leave the skin looking glowy and refreshed." Apparently, the face-crawling gastropods are fed only organic vegetables (I'm not making that up).

I found the snail story particularly ridiculous. It got full-page treatment in my local newspaper, which featured a large picture of a young, wrinkle-free model with snails on her face. The story contained a bunch of scientific-sounding jargon—pushing the idea that snail slime contained the same cocktail of "beauty-boosting" (could there be a more ambiguous term?) ingredients mentioned in the article about Katie Holmes. The only so-called experts quoted were a beauty salon employee ("Slime from snails helps remove old cells, heal the skin . . . and moisturize it") and the sales manager for the salon peddling the service. This wasn't a news story: it was an advertisement. While I am sure snail slime can help make the skin look "glowy" (*gooey* might be a more apt term), I could find no evidence to support any of the antiaging and beauty-boosting claims. In case you are interested, the sixty-minute snail treatment costs $240 and is called (again, I am not making this up) the Celebrity Escargot Course.

I realize that most of us don't take these kinds of stories too seriously. They are fun and entertaining diversions. Only a small segment of the public is willing to pay the ridiculous prices demanded by purveyors for purifying snails, placenta material, insect poison, and nightingale excrement. But these stories help to frame how we think about beauty, and they foster the illusion that celebrity status (and wealth) provides access to magically effective antiaging treatments. They make it seem as if there *is* something that can be done.

But in addition to reports of these extreme beauty treatments, there are many stories about antiaging routines that seem both less farfetched and more accessible. These are the treatments that have gone mainstream, thanks in part to celebrity endorsements. Among the most widely known are regimens involving hydration, acupuncture, coffee, and a variety of spa treatments. I'll examine all four but, first, a word about words.

Several expressions appear over and over again where beauty products are promoted. These words and phrases sound great, but they're vague, unquantifiable, and, if we are honest with ourselves, pretty meaningless. I suspect that in some instances they are used to avoid intervention by regulatory agencies because the phrasing refers to something that is tough to measure. Here are a few of my favorite nebulous antiaging and beauty terms: *radiant, revitalize, rejuvenate, vibrant, glowing, beautifying, brightening,* and *reduces the appearance of wrinkles.* If you see or hear any of these words or phrases, you can assume that you are entering a science-free zone.

Drink lots of water! I found this suggestion everywhere. Jennifer Lopez is reported to believe that it will maintain the moisture of the skin and help to delay aging. Ditto Milla Jovovich. And Jennifer Aniston allegedly drinks a hundred ounces—about twelve glasses—of water per day. As she concisely summarized in a recent interview: "I drink lots of water—water, water, water." (I hope she is never far from a toilet.) One beauty-focused publication suggests that water consumption is the absolute number-one practice you should adopt for your skin, because, well, supermodels swear by it. The article goes on to declare that we should all be drinking eight to twelve glasses a day. To this end, we should *always* carry a water bottle and, to ensure regular intake, program our smartphones to remind us to drink.

Nonsense.

There are lots of reasons to drink an adequate amount of water, obviously. Your body needs fluids. But, from a skin-care perspective, the data about its benefits is thin. Once you are properly hydrated—by drinking coffee, tea, or anything else containing H_2O—your kidneys take over. And you pee it out. The extra water does not travel to your face to make your skin look radiant or wrinkle free. A 2010 scientific review, for example, found "no proof for this recommendation" nor any evidence that drinking less water than recommended is harmful to your skin. The authors conclude that, while more research would help, it is likely "all a myth."

In fact, no scientific evidence supports one of the planet's most enduring health myths: that we all should drink eight glasses of water a day. The idea has been around for decades. Its advocates may not realize that *all* fluids, including those in fruits, vegetables, popsicles, and, yes, coffee, count toward your daily water intake. You don't, as suggested by supermodels and Jennifer Aniston, need to carry around a water bottle to ensure that you are always ideally hydrated. As noted in a report from the US Institute of Medicine of the National Academies of Science, "On a daily basis, people get adequate amounts of water from normal drinking behavior . . . and by letting their thirst guide them."

A 2013 review of available data did find that, if you are already dieting, drinking water might help with weight loss by suppressing appetite. Having a bunch of water sloshing around in your belly may, for instance, reduce your desire to inhale a Big Mac. But the association with weight loss was quite modest and was not found among individuals who were not dieting. In general, from a health and beauty perspective, little evidence supports the idea of consuming lots of water. Drink when you are thirsty.

By the way, as part of my commitment to a celebrity-informed skin-care routine, I did try, for a short spell, to drink lots of water. I heard this advice everywhere, so I thought I should give the practice a shot to see if my face started radiating. I gave it up after a few days. I had to pee constantly! How does Jen do it? I did not notice any increase in facial vibrancy as compensation for the increased trips to the urinal. Ironically, my hands started to get dry from all the post-pee hand washing. So, for me, the impact on my skin was hardly beneficial.

Cosmetic acupuncture! Many celebs enthusiastically embrace a range of complementary and alternative practices. In the context of beauty, cosmetic acupuncture, also called facial rejuvenation, is one of the most ubiquitous. It's a "Hot Celebrity Trend" (as proclaimed by Examiner. com), which, as one proponent declares, "Celebrities have approved." It has been reported that Sandra Bullock's thrice-weekly acupuncture sessions are her secret for staying young and that she has the cost of getting needles stuck in her face built into her studio contracts. Other needle-embracing celebs include Madonna, Kim Kardashian, Angelina Jolie, and the ultrahydrated Jennifer Aniston.

The alleged benefits, as outlined by the numerous clinic websites I reviewed, include the elimination of wrinkles, a reduction in double chin and sagging jowls, brightened eyes (!), improved muscle tone, elimination of oily skin, the alleviation of acne and dark spots, and improved circulation. Acupuncture is promoted as a pain free, natural, and efficacious alternative to Botox, one that will, as one website declares, bring "changes at the cellular level." Another says that results will last three to five years! So what does the evidence say about this miracle antiaging cure?

Nothing.

There appears to be little research on point. I could not find even a single well-designed study that looked at the use of acupuncture to achieve the claimed cosmetic benefits. Other researchers have confirmed that there is a dearth of good data. Given the degree to which this practice has been marketed, and the many bold and unequivocal claims made for it, you would think there would be at least some supporting research. But, as is often the case with alternative medicine, the only proofs offered are testimonials and celebrity endorsements.

Apart from the lack of evidence, there are several other reasons why we should be skeptical. First, like all uses of acupuncture, it is unclear what the mechanism of action would be. How, from a scientific perspective, could needles stuck in the face make your wrinkles and double chin go away? Many clinicians offering this service claim it increases "energy flow"—referring, I presume, to the ancient and enormously unscientific idea that there are channels, or meridians, under our skin that facilitate the flow of a life force called *qi* (pronounced "chee"). While a fun idea, it is patently absurd, given what we know about human biology. Other, slightly more plausible, mechanisms have been suggested, such as the idea that the needles cause "micro trauma," thus promoting inflammation. But, again, there is no evidence to support it.

Second, while studies show that acupuncture can be clinically useful for a range of conditions, this is usually in the treatment of subjectively assessed symptoms. For example, acupuncture is said to provide a degree of short-term relief from elbow, back, and neck pain or postsurgery nausea. Because the assessment of benefits is subjective, however, skeptics of acupuncture continue to think that these benefits can be attributed to the placebo effect. A recent commentary published in the journal *Anesthesia and Analgesia* went so far to suggest acupuncture is little more than "theatrical placebo." There is scant evidence that acupuncture can cause long-term measurable physiological changes in humans, which would be required for an acupuncture face-lift to actually work. For example, there is research on the use of acupuncture in the treatment of Bell's palsy—a relatively common disorder that causes a weakness or slight paralysis on one side of the face. Fixing this problem would require acupuncture to have a real and measurable impact in a manner not unlike what would be needed for a face-lift. A rigorous and independent review of the data found inadequate evidence to draw conclusions—which is a nice way of saying there is no evidence it works.

Third, in the well-designed studies that have shown acupuncture to be effective, the effect size is invariably small. Being stuck with needles may, for instance, provide more pain relief than a placebo does but only slightly more. So, even if we wish to be open-minded about the efficacy of cosmetic acupuncture, the most that can reasonably be hoped for is a small and short-term change. This kind of modest effect, which is the norm for the studies that have found acupuncture useful, is hardly the kind of demonstration that would transform, revitalize, and rejuvenate your face.

Putting skepticism aside, if you find lying on your back with needles in your face relaxing (I've tried it and found the sensation odd and not terribly soothing), go for it. Finding a calm moment in life is not easy. Getting an acupuncture treatment might afford you this opportunity. Or you could just take a nap.

Coffee to kill cellulite! Coffee is a pretty miraculous beverage. It has many well-documented health benefits, including reducing the risk of various diseases. There are few, if any, reasons to avoid coffee, and there may be numerous reasons to drink it. But can coffee rid your body of cellulite? Halle Berry is probably the best-known proponent of the coffee cure for this particular cosmetic conundrum. The actress regularly covers her body in coffee grounds in the belief that it will keep her skin cellulite free and, of course, radiant.

Cellulite is common. So common that it should be considered an entirely normal human trait—not something that needs treatment. About 90 percent of women—heavy, thin, tall, short—have at least some cellulite. But, despite this reality, it is one of those conditions that has been cast, often by celebrities in the service of the beauty industry, as a horrid affliction that must be eradicated, at any and all costs. (The anticellulite industry is worth billions.) The ridiculous degree to which this natural phenomenon is viewed as a blight is highlighted by the abuse celebrities take if, God forbid, a picture reveals even a hint of it on their hides. A 2011 cover of the magazine *Star* featured the headline "Stars Lose Fight with Cellulite." Inside were "8 pages of shocking photos!" of celebrities who had attempted and failed to rid themselves of cellulite, including the endlessly embattled Britney Spears. A candid 2012 picture of Scarlett Johansson on a Hawaiian beach betrayed a posterior that was less than perfect. (In fact, by any reasonable measure of beauty, she looked great.) The photograph led to a media pile-on. One online story, which had the blunt headline "Scarlett Johansson's Cellulite in a Bikini," posted dozens of pictures of the young actress, "in case you missed how much cellulite she has now." Another story printed her picture with this simple critique: "I know, look at that cellulite. Gross."

Given the satanic status of cellulite, it is no surprise that so many women (and an increasing number of men) pour money into the anticellulite industry. Indeed, it seems that a large and growing anticellulite movement has emerged, using a militarized rhetoric, as illustrated in the titles of numerous books and programs, such as *The 5 Keys to Kill Your Cellulite*, *Fight Cellulite Fast*, *Eat Right to Fight Cellulite!*, and (no surprise) Dr. Oz's televised "Secret Weapons to Fight Cellulite." Among the weapons used in the struggle are liposuction (which may, in fact, make cellulite worse), massage and toning machines (save your money), special diets (how could these possibly work?), supplements (ridiculous), and a whole bunch of creams. The coffee craze is just one of the many new trends, including new "shape wear" (aka girdles), which have, as noted in numerous uncritical articles, microfiber microencapsulated with the "slimming agent" caffeine. There are also, of course, innumerable over-the-counter creams made out of coffee, including one that promises to "banish cellulite by breaking down fat and draining away toxins." Remember, always be suspicious of claims that use the word *toxins*!

But despite the huge number of products, all the money invested in the area, the constant media coverage, and the massive demand, very few products, including coffee-infused creams and caffeinated underwear, have evidence to support their use. As summarized in an excellent 2010 review of the literature, "The best of the currently available treatments for cellulite have, at most, shown mild improvements in the appearance of cellulite, and most of these improvements are not maintained over time." Note that this skeptical and science-informed conclusion was aimed at the *best* treatments. The less science-based and fringe approaches—such as the food-oriented home remedies that call for rubbing honey, lemon juice, cayenne pepper, or apple-cider vinegar on your thighs—warrant an even higher level of suspicion. The 2010 review also found that most of the existing evidence was of poor quality, and, as a result, any claimed effectiveness for a "treatment method for cellulite reduction should be regarded as speculation." A more recent review, published in 2013, came to a similar conclusion, noting that "despite the high number of treatments for cellulite reduction available on the market, only a few scientific investigations on the efficacy of these treatments have been published."

Is there anything that can be done about cellulite? While new technologies are emerging—including lasers that zap the connective tissue that causes the bumpy appearance of cellulite—it seems the most effective approach is old-school weight loss and exercise. But while slimming down and building muscles can't hurt, even this far-from-easy approach has limitations. It is physiologically impossible to "spot reduce" or "sculpt" your body. No matter what celebrity trainers tell the world, no exercises will cause your body to lose weight or "firm" a particular body part. When it comes to cellulite treatments, start with the assumption that it doesn't work. Save your money until there is good, independent evidence to suggest long-term effectiveness.

Spa treatments and fancy facials! The spa treatment facial—that is, the application of some kind of cream made from dirt and water (aka mud), plant products, or animal parts—is one of the most common and enduring of beauty traditions. In fact, when I think "exotic beauty routine," I picture a fabulously wealthy celebrity lying on a white cot in some exclusive spa with mysterious green cream on her face and cucumbers on her eyes. It isn't hard to find well-publicized examples to support this stereotype. Angelina Jolie is said to get a treatment that uses a cream containing the eggs of Baerii sturgeon. Teri Hatcher gets red-wine baths. Mila Kunis pays thousands for diamond-and-ruby facials. And Gwyneth applies snake venom to her flawless face.

While in New York doing research for the book, I decided to check out a few of the most fashionable spas in the world, the kind of place where Mila goes for her diamond-and-ruby rubdowns. For example, the Spa at Trump in SoHo offers a range of signature treatments that are infused with gemstones. One of the spa staff, a woman named Tiffany (perfect!), showed me around the facility, noting that all their products are natural and that their oils are imported from Dubai where, apparently, the best facial oils come from. You can get a "balancing" diamond facial, because, as the spa brochure explains, "diamonds have been used since ancient times to balance the crown chakra, providing clarity, inspiration and enlightenment." Or you can opt for the "purifying" emerald treatment, because emeralds hold the energy of the Earth. But if your face requires revitalization—and, as I have learned, revitalization is *the* goal—then you need to go with the signature ruby rub. Rubies represent "the grounding principles of the root chakra," thus making the body "invigorated and vivacious." These gem treatments cost between $1,180 and $1,300, depending on the day you haul your chakra to the Trump.

I could not afford to scrub precious gems on my middle-aged—though increasingly pampered—face. Also, I don't think my chakra needed gemstone-assisted aligning. But I figured I should, at least, experience a real celebrity-worthy facial—one explicitly aimed at antiaging and beautification. To this end, I went to another well-known spa in SoHo. It was lauded by several allegedly reputable sources (i.e., online celebrity and fashion blogs) as one of the most exclusive in the city. It wasn't cheap, but the prices weren't quite as steep as those at the Trump.

The friendly staff suggested that I get a facial designed especially for men—who, I was told, make up about 30 percent of the spa's clientele. My esthetician, Jolanta, did not disappoint. She met all my preconceived spa-employee expectations. She was professional and warm and, of course, had flawless skin. She also had an exotic yet ambiguous accent that added to the calming quality of her voice. After I put on a robe and lay down on a large and exceedingly comfortable reclining chair, Jolanta went to work. For ninety minutes she applied what seemed like a dozen different creams to my face, neck, and shoulders. With soothing music playing quietly in the background (it wasn't Yanni—thank you, spa management—but it resided in that sonic genus), she explained the purpose of each phase of the treatment, including exfoliation, cleansing, tightening, and, naturally, revitalization.

My initial impression: Awesome! I totally get it. It was one of the most relaxing experiences of my life. I didn't want it to end. Each time Jolanta finished applying one product, I silently prayed that there was another to come. I left the spa feeling pleasantly light-headed and—dare I say?—pretty darn centered. But does it work? Does a facial have any true and lasting benefits? Doubtful.

I suspect that many people who go to spas don't really believe that rubies, for example, will revitalize their face. Nor do they believe that oils from Dubai have magical properties. And they don't think that a Gwyneth endorsement holds any scientific weight. Rather, they go to spas to experience what I experienced: ninety minutes of bliss. The vague and unverified notion that the treatments have a beautifying effect provides an excuse to indulge. It is a culturally endorsed and market-driven relaxation ritual. That said, according to one industry report, in 2010 there were 150 million client visits to spas in the United States alone. (The industry is huge: according to one estimate, there are approximately fourteen thousand spas in the United States, generating annual revenue of about $10 billion.) Many customers are likely paying big bucks in the belief that the treatment has tangible effects. A study of the American spa industry found that while spa goers are seeking a variety of benefits, including relaxation and escape from the hassles of life, a significant segment, a group the researchers unapologetically call hedonists, go to spas specifically for beauty benefits. They are paying to look better, younger, and revitalized. Of course, many celebrities fall into this category. They get spa facials before red-carpet events in order to look their best.

My spa treatment felt great, but did it do anything? Was I radiating? "You've got cotton stuck to your face," said my wife. Her underwhelmed response was backed up by the before-and-after pictures I took while in the changing room at the spa. No observable difference. I look like the same goof in both shots. The next day my face broke out.

It probably seems unfair to lump all spa facials into the same no-evidence-to-support-use category. There are so many different facial concoctions out there. But unless the facial cream has some pharmaceutical-grade ingredient, in which case it would need to be regulated and tested, it is not an overstatement to say there is little evidence to support the use of any spa treatment, at least if you are looking for a sustainable antiaging solution. Despite a good deal of digging, I could find almost no science to support the idea that a spa treatment will make your face radiant and wrinkle free. Many of the experts I spoke with said the same thing. Moreover, not one could think of a reason why a spa treatment would be helpful, at least from the standpoint of how a facial could, biologically speaking, work. For example, I spoke with Gary Fisher, a professor of molecular dermatology at the University of Michigan and director of the Photoaging and Aging Research Program. He noted that much of the over-the-counter market for antiaging products—which is where most spa products fall—is "driven by marketing, pseudoscience, or, in some cases, no science." I asked him specifically about the evidence for spa treatments, and he confirmed that there was little data on clinical or molecular effects of, for example, spa mud-pack treatments. "People like the feel on the face, they like the experience, but there is no science to back up benefits," he concluded. So, once again, this appears to be a largely science-free zone.

My skin-care advisor, Kirk Barber, agrees with the negative assessment of spa facials. He was not surprised that my skin had such a bad reaction to my celebrity-worthy SoHo facial. "Basic consumer folly" was Barber's blunt assessment of what is driving the whole area.

So, Does *Anything* Help Your Skin?

Given what the available evidence tells us about skin care, it seems safe to conclude that we can ignore just about all the celebrity advice, testimonials, and endorsements associated with antiaging products and practices. You aren't going to get a tangible benefit from any of the gimmicks (bird poop, leaches, snails) or, for that matter, from many of the more common antiaging practices (facials, water consumption, acupuncture). But is there anything that can be done to slow or reverse the aging process?

Let's start with prevention. In this regard, every science-informed skin expert I talked with said the same thing. Ditto all the relevant scientific literature. There is simply no dispute about the basic steps to skin health. They aren't sexy. They aren't high tech. And they are obvious and well known. In fact, Barber mentioned these items within five minutes of our initial meeting. As did almost all the other dermatologists and researchers I contacted.

First, don't smoke. As I said, obvious—but not, apparently, to the massive number of celebrities who smoke tobacco and other smokable plant products (and the 1.6 billion earthlings who currently smoke). It is deeply ironic that a community so worried about aging so often engages in one of the single most aging activities. It is easy to find photos of Sandra Bullock, Katie Holmes, Julia Roberts, Jessica Alba, Ben Affleck, Ellen DeGeneres, J-Lo, Daniel Radcliffe, Demi Moore, Drew Barrymore, Kate Winslet, Kate Beckinsale, Mila Kunis, Uma Thurman, Jennifer Aniston, and, gasp, Gwyneth with a cigarette in hand. No amount of snail slime, acupuncture, water consumption, or sheep placenta will counteract the impact of smoking. If you smoke regularly, all other antiaging and health-enhancing activities are inconsequential. Smoking *will* make you look prematurely old and wrinkled. Smokers have thinner skin, deeper wrinkles, and are more prone to various skin cancers. As noted in a review of skin care published in 2012 by University of Maryland Medical Center, "Heavy smokers in their 40s often have facial wrinkles more like those of nonsmokers in their 60s." Scary. Plus, of course, there is a good chance it will contribute to an early death.

Second, wear sunscreen. Again, obvious—but, if you believe the stats, few of us ever put the stuff on. One Canadian study, for example, found that fewer than 30 percent of those who work outside for a living wear sunscreen. One dermatologist, John R. Stanley from the University of Pennsylvania, has been quoted as saying that "sun protection is the single most important thing to ensure your skin looks good for a long time. All the other things you could do to your skin are so minor compared to sun protection." Research confirms this assertion. A recent study, published in the *Annals of Internal Medicine* in 2013, followed more than nine hundred randomly selected adults for 4.5 years. The researchers found that the skin of the group assigned to use sunscreen on a daily basis aged 24 percent less than the group that was allowed to use sunscreen on a discretionary basis. It should be noted that this benefit was observed during a period of fewer than five years. Wearing sunscreen for longer would produce an even greater discrepancy between those who use sunscreen and those who don't. You should, of course, take other steps to reduce sun exposure, including wearing a hat.

Third, sleep. This one is perhaps not so obvious. But if good skin is a priority, get your z's. A growing body of literature supports the importance of sleep for health generally. Research has found that humans are good at picking up facial cues that indicate people who are sleep deprived. A 2010 study, for example, found that people who do not get enough sleep are rated as less attractive, less healthy, and (naturally) more tired than those who are appropriately rested. Research also hints that a lack of sleep may cause wrinkles. A 2013 study done at Case Western Reserve University School of Medicine followed sixty women and found that those who got poor-quality sleep had increased signs of aging, including fine lines, uneven pigmentation, a slackening of the skin, and reduced skin elasticity. Other studies have demonstrated a strong connection between a lack of sleep and an increased risk for a range of ailments, including obesity and diabetes. Kids who go to bed late, for example, are more likely to have a high BMI. In fact, a 2010 analysis of all relevant research found that poor sleep was a "significant predictor of death." As I said, get your z's!

Many of us aren't getting nearly enough sleep. The US Centers for Disease Control and Prevention reports that approximately one-third of the population averages fewer than six hours a night. (Adults should get between seven and nine.) That means there are more than forty million Americans whose skin is prematurely aging as a result of poor sleeping habits. Forget the spa. Forget the bird poop. Go to bed!

Fourth and fifth: eat a healthy diet and exercise regularly. These last two are tricky. I love this advice and intuitively believe it to be true. Also, it makes sense that if you are living a healthy lifestyle—and diet and exercise are critical to achieving maximum health—this might be reflected in how your skin looks. Some experts suggest that exercise increases blood flow, which, the argument goes, is good for the skin. Makes sense. Others suggest that a healthy diet provides the skin with all the necessary nutrients. This also makes sense. But I could only find a few relevant clinical studies to support these sensible suggestions. A study of more than five hundred women in the United Kingdom, China, and Spain found that an unhealthy lifestyle—by which the researchers meant smoking, eating poorly, not exercising, getting too much sun—added a staggering 10.4 years to your facial age. Similarly, a 2012 study found that the consumption of olive oil and healthy diet habits were associated with reduced skin aging. Finally, research presented in 2014 by a team from McMaster University found that exercise seems to keep skin healthier. It may even help to reverse the aging process. The researchers took skin biopsies from the research participants and found that those who exercised regularly had healthier skin with more youthful characteristics than those who did not get regular exercise.

So, given the logic of this advice and the emerging evidence, I am inclined to fully embrace the diet-and-exercise prescription for good skin. Long term, a healthy lifestyle has an impact.

Smoke Signals and Tanning Tales

"I exercise all the time! One, two hours a day . . . sometimes more. Fitness is key. It depends on the part, but you need to work hard. You have no idea. Everyone [in Hollywood] is working out."

I am sitting across from a young actor on the patio of a cafe in West Hollywood. He is slim and ridiculously handsome—the kind of handsome that makes you hate him until you discover what a nice guy he is, and then you like him too much. While not famous, he is a working actor who knows the business well. He has appeared in Hollywood movies and on popular TV shows. He has just finished playing the lead in a film shot in Germany. He is telling me about what he must do to remain competitive in the ridiculously competitive world of acting. And while he outlines the importance of diet ("the cliché is true: the camera does put on pounds," he says) and exercise, the young, attractive, hardworking actor smokes a cigarette. He does this without any apparent recognition of the irony implicit in the behavior. No mention of some bad addiction he just can't shake. Nothing he says suggests that I might find his words and actions incongruous. And he really seems to be enjoying the damn thing. It is his second within less than an hour.

Until I started researching this book, I almost never saw young people smoking. Sometimes I catch one of my students sheepishly sneaking a smoke outside the law school. But they always look ashamed. Addiction isn't fun, their slumped frames say, especially when it is forty degrees below zero outside. But among actors, smoking seems to be the norm. I might be wrong about this. I can't find any scientific data to support my impression that almost all actors smoke. And, thanks to effective antismoking campaigns, the media tend to avoid publishing pictures of celeb smokers. Indeed, many publicists actively work to keep the smoking habits of their clients out of the press. But my experiences in Hollywood and New York sure support the "actors smoke" cliché. (As do the reliable "data" I collected from celebrity gossip websites such as IMDb, TMZ, and Lainey Gossip.) I appreciate that many smoke as a means of controlling appetite. As noted, the pressure to stay slim, especially for women, is ridiculous. Still, it is odd to see—in this antismoking era—so many embrace the habit.

Let's set the record straight: smoking is an idiotic weight-loss strategy. In addition to the good chance it will kill you (as succinctly summarized by the World Health Organization, "Tobacco kills up to half of its users"), smoking is associated with eventual weight gain, insulin resistance, and an unhealthy distribution of fat—among other nasty things. As noted in a 2008 review of the relevant data, over the long haul, the "data suggest that smoking may not help to control weight. . . . If anything, smoking (in particular, heavy smoking) seems related to weight gain." Also, unless you plan to smoke yourself into the grave, you will also put on a lot of weight when you quit (which, by the way, will likely take seven to eight attempts). A 2012 study published in the *British Medical Journal* found that, on average, people gain about eleven pounds after quitting smoking. (Note: despite the weight gain, quitting is *still* a good idea!) From a weight-control perspective, smoking is doubly bad: Start smoking, gain weight. Quit smoking, gain weight.

What I find particularly fascinating are the dual (and always unspoken) messages emanating from the celebrity universe. Message one: be youthful and sexy. Message two: smoke. These messages are in complete contradiction. It is a contradiction for the actors trying to stay youthful and for the public who are influenced by celebrity culture.

I am not *blaming* the handsome actor for the messed-up messaging. He is caught by the paradox too. But we shouldn't underplay the influence of pop culture on smoking behavior. Research has consistently shown that the smoking behavior of celebrities can have an influence on smoking uptake. (My West Hollywood cafe companion looked so darn cool while inhaling that I thought about asking for a cig.) A study published in the *American Journal of Public Health*, for example, concluded, "Smoking by movie stars can play an important role in encouraging female adolescents to start smoking." Other research has found that smoking in movies can lead adolescents to take up the habit. One study from 2005 found "strong empirical evidence indicates that smoking in movies increases adolescent smoking initiation" and went on to recommend that movies with smoking should always receive an R rating. The situation is improving. Fewer teenagers are smoking, at least in developed nations.

The amount of smoking in movies and on TV has decreased since the mid-2000s. Still, there are ample recent examples of popular culture's negative influence. The popular and critic-revered show *Mad Men* helped to boost the sale of cigarettes, particularly the iconic Lucky Strike brand often featured on the program. Sales of the cigarettes were twenty-three billion packs in 2007, when the show first aired. In 2012 their sales reached thirty-three billion packs. Apparently, there are even drinking and smoking games associated with the show. Participants must drink and smoke when the characters do so.

Gwyneth made an off-the-cuff comment that she has the occasional smoke because the indulgence helps her to kick back and chill or, as she said, allows her "just the right amount of naughty"—and thus helps her look vibrant. This is so ludicrous (and, from a public health perspective, so harmful) that it is hard not to be a bit angry with the actor, particularly as she has set herself up as the paragon of healthy living. It is not as if it was an incidental comment. She runs a health and lifestyle business, and this is presented as health advice.

OF COURSE, SMOKING isn't the only area where there is a bizarre conflict with the dominant "look young!" message flowing from the celebrity universe. Another is in the realm of tanning and sun exposure. As I have noted, absolutely every expert agrees that unprotected exposure to the sun's rays is one of the worst things you can do for your skin. Combine tanning with smoking and you are destined to look prematurely old. Guaranteed. And yet, many in the youth-obsessed world of celebrities promote the practice.

In 2013, *British Cosmopolitan* quoted Gwyneth as saying: "We're human beings and the sun is the sun—how can it be bad for you? I think we should all get sun and fresh air. . . . I don't think anything that is natural can be bad for you." Putting aside the absurd idea that all things natural are healthy (consider, for example, arsenic, black widow venom, tar sand, earthquakes, gravity pulling you toward the ground at terminal velocity), the idea that we should all be tanning is so clearly wrong that it makes you wonder what Gwyneth was thinking.

The "pro-tan" subculture—yes, this really exists, as evidenced by the many websites devoted to the maintenance of a bronze glow—loved Gwyneth's endorsement and repeated it again and again. For example, the president of a tanning advocacy group (I imagine these guys hanging in a cloud-shrouded castle with the tobacco, junk food, and gambling advocates) called Smart Tan opined thus: "Hopefully Paltrow's advice will translate into other public figures taking a more sensible approach to sun care." By a "sensible approach," I don't think the boss of Smart Tan—a brand name the *New England Journal of Medicine* called oxymoronic— was referring to avoiding sun exposure.

Virtually any science-informed expert will tell you there is no such thing as a healthy tan. That is, in fact, the opening sentence of a World Health Organization report. The American Skin Association, the Skin Cancer Foundation, Health Canada, the Canadian Cancer Society, and the UK National Health Service, among many other health-focused orga- nizations, all have publications that repeat this axiom. Why the hostility, you might wonder? The answer is made explicit in the WHO document: "A suntan may be cosmetically desirable, but in fact it is nothing but a sign that your skin has been damaged and has attempted to protect itself."

Not only does tanning age the skin; it also is a serious health risk. Skin cancer is on the rise. It is the most common form of cancer in North America and one of the most common cancer diagnoses among those younger than thirty. A 2012 study in *Mayo Clinic Proceedings* found that since the mid-1970s the rates of melanoma, a deadly form of skin cancer, grew by 800 percent (yep, *800*) among women and 400 percent among men. A 2010 study published in the *Archives of Dermatology* con- cluded that skin cancer is now an "underrecognized epidemic." And the US Centers for Disease Control and Prevention (CDC) recently cau- tioned that skin cancer is an urgent public health problem and said that "if current trends continue, one in five Americans will get skin cancer in their lifetime." And yet, despite this grim reality, numerous studies have also found that tanning is on the rise, especially among the young. One study of US college students found that a shocking 60 percent had used a tanning booth in 2013 and that 83 percent thought that having a tan was very or somewhat important.

While the developed world's affinity for a "healthy tan," which really took off in the mid-twentieth century, has myriad sources—including a shift from its association with the poor and the working class—there seems little doubt that celebrity culture has played an important role. Legend has it that the tanning fad started when the fashion icon Coco Chanel was photographed with a tan she inadvertently obtained while on a Mediterranean cruise. Though this story may be apocryphal, a good deal of solid research supports the role of celebrities in promoting tanning. Nina G. Jablonski, a biological anthropologist from Pennsylvania State University, has noted that tanning practices "were instigated and are maintained by celebrities, whose images are widely propagated by the media." She has also suggested that highly imitated female celebrities, such as Britney Spears and Paris Hilton, "have done much to promote both real and fake tanning, giving much impetus to booth-and-bottle, look-good-feel-good promotions at tanning establishments." Many studies support Jablonski's view. Another study, published in 2012, found that people who watch reality television beauty shows are "significantly more likely to use tanning beds and to tan outdoors than those who do not." And a 2013 study of college students found that "the glamorization of a 'healthy tan'" was a key factor in the increase in risky sun-tanning behaviors and negative attitudes toward sun protection.

There are, to be fair, a few signs that pop culture portrayals about tanning and the importance of sunscreen are evolving. Actors such as Victoria Beckham and Nicole Kidman now favor a more natural look. Still, the dominant pop-culture message remains very pro-tan. As noted in a study from Australia that examined popular magazines, the "implicit messages about sun protection in popular Australian women's magazines contradict public health messages concerning skin cancer prevention."

By the way, just so there is no confusion, using a tanning bed is *not* a safe, or even a safer, way to tan. Some public health agencies, such as the

CDC, have bluntly stated that tanning beds cause cancer. Shockingly, using a tanning bed before you're thirty-five increases your chance of getting cancer by 75 percent. It is no surprise, therefore, that the World Health Organization has classified tanning devices as carcinogenic.

The paradoxes that flow from the tension between the obsession with a youthful appearance and the aging effects of sun exposure and tanning are made all the more bizarre because research tells us that the public still equates a bronze complexion with health, vitality, and youthfulness, even though, from a biological perspective, it represents skin damage, decay, and accelerated aging. As with so many activities, people eventually come to regret their embrace of practices done for the sole purpose of vanity. A recent study out of the United Kingdom found that many adults deeply regret sunbathing in their youth—and 40 percent blame their parents for not warning them about the long-term consequences!

AFTER REREADING THE preceding rant about smoking and sun exposure, I realized two things.

First, I come off as an alarmist, self-righteous killjoy. In reality, I know that not everyone who gets a tan will get skin cancer (though the relationship between smoking and ill health is a bit more certain, verging on one to one). It's possible that my vehemence is a defensive response, attributable to my having done a pretty bad job for the last five decades of taking care of my own skin. Until I got skin-care advice from Kirk Barber and Marie, I almost never wore sunscreen, even though I have regularly spent hours and hours in outdoor activities, such as cycling. I have frequently burned my skin and worried little. (Burning your skin is another risk factor for skin cancer.) I have also enjoyed the "healthy tan" that I developed as summer progressed and felt that it projected a youthful energy. I was wrong. Second, I have ignored one of the most important aspects of the aging story, genetics. The state of my facial pores and wrinkles likely has absolutely nothing to do with my lifelong beauty regimen (that is, the occasional use of plain soap) but is the result, at least in part, of some genetic predisposition. Recent research has shown that genetics plays an important role in how skin ages. This is one reason ethnicity is an important predictor of both how skin will age and skin-cancer risk. And there is also a big difference between males and females, which is also, of course, genetic. Male skin, for example, is much thicker than the female skin and thus shows signs of aging more slowly.

Indeed, the amount of sun exposure, your smoking habits, and your genes probably account for more than 90 percent of the factors that determine how your skin will age. While you can modify the first two, you can't pick your parents. Genetics is luck. And, of course, many celebrities got very, very lucky. The fact that individuals who have won the beauty-gene lottery are setting universal beauty standards is a bit like using NBA power forwards to inspire people to endeavor to be tall.

Reversing the Aging Process?

There is universal agreement on the basic steps to prevent premature aging. But what if the damage is already done? Or what if you simply want to look younger and reduce wrinkles? For the purpose of this analysis, I am setting aside the whole concept of aging gracefully and the widespread obsession with looking young. These are important points that deserve critical attention, but what I am interested in here is what the available evidence tells us about what, if anything, can be done to make a dramatic change in our appearance. To explore this topic, I thought it best to go to one of the epicenters of the celebrity-driven youth culture: Beverly Hills.

"I was street smart, but unfortunately the street was Rodeo Drive," Carrie Fisher has famously said about the notorious California drag. And anyone who has spent even a small amount of time walking its sidewalks instantly gets the joke. It is a strange place—a mix of fashion runway, over-the-top luxury shops, and Vegas-style architecture. It is an unapologetic salute to consumerism and opulence. The pedestrians on Rodeo seem to come in three discrete varieties: the tourist (distinctive features: shorts, T-shirt, and sneakers); the local businessperson (tan, smartphone at the ready, expensive suit/dress, and even more expensive shoes); and the species at the top of the hierarchy, the serious shopper (dark tan, big jewelry/watch, sports car/SUV, and, especially if past a certain age, a surgically enhanced facade).

As I stroll the street, looking mostly like I belong squarely in the first category, I wonder if the facial appearance of this last group is the result of the abundance of antiaging physicians—dermatologists, plastic surgeons—on the streets that run parallel to Rodeo Drive. Or is the reverse true? Is the abundance of the doctors the result of the presence of this dominant Rodeo class? A complex symbiotic relationship exists, no doubt, but I suspect it is mostly the latter. The large number of people with the financial resources to pay for these specialists' services is likely the main reason so many world-renowned antiaging experts are clustered here.

Dr. Rhonda Rand is one of these experts. As I wait to chat with her about effective antiaging strategies, I peruse the product posters that cover the walls of her waiting room. All the advertisements include pictures of ridiculously youthful-looking women and a range of rejuvenation promises: wrinkle reduction, skin tightening, and, as offered by one poster, "youthfulness that is uniquely you."

Rand is a respected dermatologist who has practiced in Beverly Hills for almost thirty years. She trained with Kirk Barber at Harvard and teaches at UCLA. Though the rules around patient confidentiality prevent her from mentioning or even hinting at any names, it is common knowledge that she has, like many of the physicians around the Rodeo hub, many well-known celebrity clients. Rand knows dermatology and she knows Hollywood. She and her physician colleagues are on the front line of the celebrity culture. They help to create the faces that create the broader social expectations of beauty and youth. "Everyone [in this city] wants to look young," she tells me. "For many it is an expectation, part of the job. They need to look good for the camera. It is a youth culture. And not just for actors. Writers, directors, grips . . . there is a lot of pressure on everyone." Given this pressure, I am curious to learn what can be done. Are there any products and procedures proven to make skin look younger and less wrinkled?

The Big Three

While aging is a complex process that involves many biological changes, most aging (i.e., wrinkles) results from a breakdown in the substances that give skin its structure (collagen) and strength (elastin). Also, as we age, our skin gets thinner, our oil glands become less effective, and our cells don't divide as quickly. Any treatment that is going to have a measurable impact must deal with at least a few of these issues, particularly the collagen problem. Indeed, a wonderful review written for the *Archives of Dermatology* (Gary Fisher was the lead author) noted that the available evidence tells us that "collagen fragmentation"—a natural part of getting old but one that is accelerated by such factors as exposure to the sun (photoaging)—is the primary culprit in the aging of skin.

"What can be done?" I ask Rand. "What really works to reverse the aging process?"

You will note that my inquiry focuses on undoing the damage, not on surgically altering your face. I want to know if anything will modify the biological processes I have just outlined. And to my surprise (I went into this investigation with a deep, BIEB-informed skepticism) there are—roughly, as there are a few other procedures and creams that could fall into these categories—three reasonable and evidence-based options.

Now, I don't want this section of the book to serve as promotion for the antiaging industry. I am not thrilled that we live in a world where this is a rapidly growing, multibillion-dollar industry. But here goes. I will be brief.

Retinoids. "Retinoids are simply *the* gold standard," Rand tells me. "There is lots of evidence to support their use." Retinoids are a derivative of vitamin A and include a range of compounds such as retinol and retinoic acid. Many studies have shown that products that contain a sufficiently high concentration of these compounds, and usually applied as a topical agent, will stimulate the growth of collagen and improve the appearance of aging skin. But, as a 2011 article in *Clinical Pharmacology and Therapeutics* noted, while the results are objectively measurable, they "can be subtle and occur over fairly long periods of time." So, though effective, retinoids (and other emerging compounds that may produce biological changes, such as products containing vitamin C) are far from a magical solution to aging skin.

Resurfacing. The next broad category of effective procedures can best be thought of as "controlled wounding," a term Gary Fisher used to describe the techniques used to ablate (i.e., remove or destroy) old skin in order to stimulate the growth of new, less wrinkled skin. Rand referred to a radiofrequency technique, but the use of various forms of lasers is probably the most common and studied approach. As with retinoids, the data are solid. Resurfacing, as it is sometimes called, reduces wrinkles. Rand told me she had used this technique on her own neck. She looks pretty amazing. There are a couple of caveats to keep in mind when considering this approach. You likely need to actually create a wound. That's how, from a biological perspective, the procedure works. So any resurfacing techniques that are minimally invasive are of more questionable cosmetic value (though some evidence suggests that aggressive microderm abrasion *may* stimulate collagen production). Also, the recovery time can be significant.

Fillers. Finally, there are all the different fillers that can be injected into your face. Initially, I had no idea that these approaches could actually cause a biological change. I thought they were simply used to fill in the wrinkles. Indeed, when Rand first mentioned this approach, she said that it is sometimes used to make the faces of hyperthin actors look less skeletal. But studies have found that fillers, which can use collagen and hyaluronic acid, stretch the skin and, as a result, stimulate collagen production.

Other emerging, but as yet unproven, technologies may provide treatment for aging skin. Stem cell research may lead to some kind of breakthrough (clinical applications are likely years, perhaps decades, away), and a few other antioxidants *may* be beneficial, but, to date, I think it is fair to say that retinoids, resurfacing, and fillers capture what's most effective and available. I could go into more detail about the risks associated with some of them—for example, retinoids can be hard on the skin. But the important point is that there are, despite the billions of dollars spent and all the noise and marketing, only a handful of effective approaches. Of course, these are the strategies celebrities frequently use to maintain their mugs.

Botox

I am sure you have been thinking, *But what about Botox?*

It works. If used properly, it works quite well. It's safe. It is huge. Everyone in Hollywood uses it. Some use it way too much. You don't need to hear more from me on the subject.

Over-the-Counter = Undertested

"Whatever it is, it should probably be prescription strength," Rand said when I told her about my new beauty routine. "In many [over-the-counter] products, the dosage is so low it doesn't do anything."

Like Gary Fisher, she is skeptical about the effectiveness of over-the-counter antiaging products. (And, by the way, like Carrie Fisher, no relation, Rand is also fully aware of the strangeness of her locale. "It's hard, but you've got to put this stuff in perspective," she said with a laugh when asked how people should respond to the youth culture pressure flowing from Hollywood.) Rand's doubt seems entirely justified. A 2012 review of the available evidence associated with over-the-counter (OTC) topical antiaging products found that almost no good research is available. The authors' conclusion is worth quoting at length because it does a nice job of underscoring how absurd it is that a multibillion-dollar industry, one that is purportedly based on cutting-edge science, generally has no good science to back up its promises (the BIEB is a strong social force!).

Overall, there is a great necessity for more rigorous studies of OTC skin-care products. This is especially imperative because these products comprise such a significant percentage of the enormous cosmeceutical industry. The average woman in the United States uses at least twenty-five products containing hundreds of ingredients on her skin daily. Few of these OTC products, which may cost hundreds of dollars, have been subjected to rigorous controlled trials of efficacy.

Not only are many of the ingredients in OTC products unproven, when they do (allegedly) include a potentially effective ingredient, like retinol, the dosage is so low or the form of the product is so unclear that the clinical value remains questionable. Key terms are thrown around in marketing as a way to make the products seem scientifically legitimate. Also, many chemicals used in these products, including, for example, the antioxidant vitamin C, are relatively unstable. Maintaining the chemical in a pharmaceutically usable form is not easy: simply stuffing it in a jar won't do the trick. As a 2012 paper noted on the use of ascorbic acid (aka: vitamin C) as an antiaging agent, "Unfortunately, it seems, many products in the market still fail even the most rudimentary [stability] analysis."

Given these realities, it is safe to assume that almost all over-the-counter products, particularly any that seem too good to be true, are probably not worth your money or time. You can ignore celebrity endorsements, no matter how enthusiastic and heartfelt. Gwyneth recently used her Goop website to endorse a sonic-infusion thingy, which an evidence-free (naturally) article on the product in the *Daily Mail* reported "infuse[s] the outer layers of the skin with anti-aging sea serum." This is utter nonsense, but that didn't stop Gwyneth from saying she has "been obsessed with mine ever since I started using it. I've seen a real difference in my skin."

This leads me to an interesting paradox. When I told people about my research on celebrities and beauty, almost everyone said they knew it was all bull. I don't recall a single person who said something like "Really?

I was so sure Gwyneth's sonic sea-serum injector really worked. How disappointing. I want my money back!" People claim to be aware that antiaging products won't work and that celebrity endorsements are absurd. But despite this, they keep on spending thousands of dollars on these products and using them daily. It is a huge and growing industry. Some people seem to spend money on this stuff simply because it is expensive. During a panel convened to discuss the lack of evidence and unregulated nature of the cosmeceutical industry at the annual meeting of the American Society of Cosmetic Dermatology and Aesthetic Surgery, it was noted there is now a $700 moisturizer. But, as one panelist observed, "there may be no difference between it and a $10 one. But people will pay $700 because it's $700."

There is a peculiar paradox apparent in what we think and what we do when it comes to these items. A Canadian study published in 2010 confirmed that the main reason women buy beauty products is, no surprise here, to maintain a youthful-looking appearance. The women in the study equated looking better with general well-being. And they equated looking younger with feeling younger. But even though achieving tangible benefits was their stated goal, only 3 percent of the more than three hundred women in the study thought over-the-counter antiaging products actually worked! As the authors noted, "Women, on one hand, questioned the effectiveness of anti-aging products (and felt they were overpriced) but, on the other hand, still purchased and used them."

Amy Muise, the lead author of the study and a social psychologist from the University of Toronto, told me she was surprised by the strength of these ironic results. "Perhaps they are not sure how effective these products are but figure it can't hurt and may help a little bit or be preventive of future aging. . . . Even women who find these products gimmicky, or want to embrace natural aging, cannot escape these deeply embedded cultural norms."

Before I leave Rand's 90210 office, I ask her what she would do to improve my aging face. Is it a lost cause? She moves a bit closer, leans in, and her expression immediately changes. She is no longer looking at me. She is now *examining* me. Just a few seconds later she has a verdict:

she'd consider filler on my cheeks and perhaps some Botox between my eyebrows. Given how quickly she made this assessment, I wonder if she was deliberating my many imperfections throughout our conversation. It must be an occupational hazard, particularly in Beverly Hills, where no expense is spared and there is always *something* that can be done.

She offered no comment on my repulsive pore situation.

Reassessment

Nine months after my visit with Dr. Rand, I show up for my dermatologist appointment to have the condition of my skin reassessed. I have been using the products provided at my visit to the skin-care clinic in Calgary relatively faithfully during the past year. I say "relatively" because it is difficult to get all the products through airport security and, as a result, I do the full routine only when I am at home. Still, this is the most, by far, that I have ever done for my skin. I have exfoliated, moisturized, cleansed, decongested, tightened, and protected for the better part of a year. The products used in the routine were expensive and the commitment of time considerable. So are there any measurable improvements? Did all that pampering achieve anything?

Before I proceed, I must report a bit of a twist to my investigative strategy. Instead of going back to the original Calgary clinic, I decided to go to a *different* dermatologist, one who has no idea that this is an "after" test. This strategy, or so my thinking goes, will help to ensure a relatively objective assessment. If my skin has improved, it should be noticeable by any skin-care expert. I simply tell the staff at the new clinic that I am curious about the condition of my skin, which is absolutely true, and that I want to know what can be done to improve it.

The new clinic, which will remain nameless, has the identical *Star Trek* machine that was used to assess my skin in Calgary one year ago. The clinic staff takes pictures of my face just as the first staff did. To be fair, I suppose there may be calibration differences between the machines. But any significant difference, one that would be visible to the outside world—which is, after all, the whole point—should be detectable.

The results? Not impressive. Compared to people of my age and ethnicity, I'm told, my skin actually got *worse* on four of the eight assessment criteria, including texture and the all-important wrinkle category. (Just so there is no confusion about how underwhelming these results are, I am being compared to a cohort of individuals of the same age.) My skin scores are about the same (within a few percentage points) on two of the criteria, including pores. The only area that shows significant improvement is the amount of porphyrins on my skin, which is a by-product of bacteria. That is to say, my skin is now cleaner, which is no surprise. I have been doing a lot of scrubbing!

After the dermatologist finishes reviewing my skin analysis, he recommends several over-the-counter antiaging products, at a cost of more than $500 for a six-month supply. These products and potions will dramatically improve my skin situation, or so he promises.

Thanks but no thanks. I've heard that before. Back to ordinary soap and water.

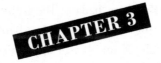

Pamela Anderson's Breasts

Few would argue with the proposition that many cosmetic surgery trends have roots in celebrity culture. One could put forward a pretty convincing argument that *all* cosmetic surgery trends—big breasts, perky noses, butt implants (this is a thing)—have roots in celebrity culture, but we don't need to go that far. The point I am positing here is simply that celebrity images play a significant role in how all of us, men and women, want to look and, perhaps more important, in our never-ending dissatisfaction with our current appearance. As I have already mentioned (and will mention again because it can't be mentioned enough when you are writing about this topic), I fully appreciate that the relationship between celebrity culture and public perceptions and desires is complex. Indeed, there is a huge body of academic literature on this issue, and I will touch on some of it in the pages that follow. Of course, we can't say that celebrity culture is 100 percent responsible for a particular trend: it isn't a direct causal effect. Jennifer Aniston doesn't drive to people's homes and force them to cut their hair in a certain way. Still, we know celebrity culture plays a significant role.

This comes under the heading of anecdotal evidence, but I once spent much more than I should have on a watch because I saw David Beckham wearing it in an interview. He looked pretty darn hip. I am wearing it as I type these words, but I think I am projecting a vibe that is more midlife mistake than Beckham badass. The influence that celebs have had on the mainstreaming of tattoos—again, thanks, Mr. Beckham—is perhaps a better example. A number of academics have observed how celebrities have changed the public's perception of tattoos, which once were viewed as a blue-collar phenomenon and now are widely accepted as a white-collar trend with a degree of aesthetic and cultural legitimacy. As suggested by the sociologist Mary Kosut, an expert on the place of tattoos in popular culture, the "celebrity tattoo phenomenon" has "elevate[d] tattoos' cultural status." Remarkably, 21 percent of Americans now have a tattoo. For people aged eighteen to twenty-five, the figure is 36 percent, and more than 40 percent for those aged twenty-six to forty, the Gen Xers. Thanks in large part to celebrities and increased media coverage, the tattoo industry now is worth more than $2.3 billion.

I selected cosmetic surgery as an example of celebrity influence because it is a relatively extreme act (you are, after all, having someone cut into your flesh to alter your appearance). Like a tattoo, surgery isn't easy to reverse. It is a big decision that involves numerous steps, including the involvement of licensed and formally regulated health professionals who have a legal obligation to do what is in the best interest of their patients. It is not, in other words, a trivial matter for celebrity culture to impinge on the world of cosmetic surgery.

Incidentally, this discussion is not just relevant to women. In 2011, 9 percent of surgical and nonsurgical cosmetic procedures in the United States were conducted on men, according to the American Society for Aesthetic Plastic Surgery—a 121 percent increase since 1997.

ONE OF THE fastest-growing forms of plastic surgery is an arm lift. This is exactly what it sounds like: surgery (often liposuction) to make your arms look slimmer. Since 2001 the popularity of this procedure in the United States has grown 4,378 percent. Crazy. More than fifteen thousand people, 98 percent of them women, had this surgery performed in 2012. What caused this love affair with the upper limb? A 2012 survey by the American Society of Plastic Surgeons found increasing attention was being paid to female celebrity arms. Michelle Obama has the most admired arms (41 percent), followed closely by Jennifer Aniston (29 percent). Other celebs with influential appendages include Jessica Biel (13 percent), Kelly Ripa (13 percent), and Demi Moore (11 percent). (Wasn't Gwyneth on the list? Recount!)

And then there's Kate Middleton's nose. According to data provided by the UK plastic surgery industry, requests for the princess's nose tripled in 2012. And the royal snout seems equally popular in the United States. "New York Women Rushing to Get the Kate Middleton Nose," noted a 2013 headline from the *New York Daily News*. "I love the shape and size of Kate Middleton's nose and just knew I had to have it," a twenty-six-year-old told the paper. For men, an increasingly large part of the cosmetic surgery market, the desired looks include Ryan Gosling's lips and Jude Law's cheeks.

Studies have found that media exposure, including TV and magazines, is associated with an increased anxiety about both aging and body dissatisfaction, two factors that contribute to decisions to get cosmetic surgery. In addition, researchers have determined that the use of cosmetic surgery by celebrities normalizes and trivializes the process, thus increasing acceptability. Other studies have found a more direct relationship between celebrities and cosmetic surgery. For example, a study published in 2011 measured the attitudes of young adults toward celebrities. The research found that feeling a connection to celebrities, particularly celebs with attractive bodies, was a strong predictor of future cosmetic surgery. The authors conclude that the "findings present compelling evidence for a strong association between celebrity worship and a willingness to undergo cosmetic surgery." Another study, published in 2009, examined the impact of TV shows that feature cosmetic surgery, including shows such as ABC's *Extreme Makeover*, Fox's *The Swan*, and E!'s *Doctor 90210*. The study, which involved about two thousand college students, was definitive but predictable: "Viewership of reality cosmetic surgery shows was significantly related to more favorable cosmetic surgery attitudes, perceived pressure to have cosmetic surgery, past attainment of a cosmetic procedure, a decreased fear of surgery, as well as overall body dissatisfaction, media internalization, and disordered eating."

It is worth noting that the impact of celebrity, and especially Hollywood culture, is global. As one Beverly Hills plastic surgeon told the *Atlantic* about his work in Dubai, "They say, 'I want a Beyonce butt, I want a J-Lo butt, I want a Kim Kardashian butt,' and it's amazing to think the same things I'm doing here, I'm doing over there." South Korea has the highest per-capita rate of plastic surgery in the world—according to some estimates more than 20 percent of the population has gone under the knife. With the rise in the international profile of Korean popular culture—often called K-pop—there has been a concomitant rise in cosmetic procedures, including radical physical alterations, such as jaw surgery. The most sought-after attributes are those of South Korean celebrities. These include a V-shaped jaw, big eyes, and a delicate nose. To get an appreciation of the preferred look, check out the dancers on the YouTube video for Psy's massive hit, "Gangnam Style." Most unsettlingly, it appears that a significant percentage of the people getting surgery in Korea are teenagers. One story about the phenomenon reported that 20 percent of one well-known surgeon's patients were younger than twenty and that most requested "a certain feature of K-pop stars."

In 2013 the UK Royal College of Surgeons recommended that surgeons avoid telling patients that cosmetic surgery will make them look better. At first, this seems counterproductive, comparable to instructing deodorant vendors to tell customers that their product will have no effect on their BO. But the goal of the college is to ensure that patients' expectations remain realistic. It even goes so far as to suggest that when discussing the likely outcomes of cosmetic procedures, surgeons should avoid using descriptive terms such as *nicer* and *better* and instead use more neutral words, such as *bigger* and *smaller*. This policy appears to be the result of two trends: the increasing popularity of cosmetic surgery and the growing desire of many individuals to look like, or acquire a particular feature of, a celebrity.

Obviously, people have myriad reasons for getting cosmetic surgery. Not all are driven by popular culture representations of physical beauty.

Many are simply striving for what they perceive to be physical normality (though those perceptions are likely mediated, at least in part, by celebrity images) or believe that a particular feature may be socially problematic. For many, perhaps most, cosmetic surgery is a perfectly sensible decision, the result of thoughtful reflection and appropriate clinical consultation. Indeed, there is reason to think that the majority of individuals are pleased with the results of surgery. A 2013 study from Germany, for example, followed more than five hundred first-time surgery patients. While a not insignificant number of the patients, about 12 percent, had unrealistic expectations (such as believing that "all my problems will be solved" and "I'll be a completely new person"), the vast majority said they had achieved their desired goals, at least in the short term (the study lasted one year).

David Sarwer is a psychologist at the University of Pennsylvania School of Medicine and a renowned expert on body image, particularly as it relates to cosmetic surgery. Sarwer wonders about the long-term effects, especially of those decisions influenced by celebrity-mediated norms of beauty. "Patients often articulate their desires in a definitive manner. But will they feel the same way in five years about breast implants? Views change." Sarwer's comments are pertinent for two reasons. First, recent research tells us that we are terrible at predicting how we will feel in the future—we all think we know what our future selves will value and how we will think—but we are usually wrong. A study published in 2013 in the journal *Science* used data from more than nineteen thousand individuals and "found consistent evidence to indicate that people underestimate how much they will change in the future, and that doing so can lead to suboptimal decisions." We can all think of personal examples of this phenomenon. If he had had his way, the twenty-year-old me would have had "The Clash" tattooed across his back. (On second thought, that's a bad example. That still sounds pretty cool.) In the context of cosmetic surgery, the implications are obvious.

And this leads to the second reason Sarwer's caution seems sensible. Celebrity fads are, inevitably and perhaps increasingly, transient. The popularity of Kate Middleton's nose seems destined to fade, at least to some degree. But unlike other fashion trends—from high-waisted bell-bottoms to low-rider skinny jeans—a fashion fad that is the result of a surgical procedure is not easy to reverse. And any alteration that is tethered to a particular celebrity-driven look is bound to result in a degree of long-term disappointment.

IT IS DIFFICULT to overstate the popularity of the beachwear-centric TV show *Baywatch*, even in reruns. By some estimates, at its peak it was watched each week by more than a billion people in about 140 countries. To put that in perspective, about ten million people watched the final episode of *Breaking Bad*—which is one one-hundredth of the regular audience of *Baywatch*. *The Guinness Book of World Records* declared it the most-watched program on the planet. And it produced one of the most famous individuals of all time (I'll support this claim in a moment): Pamela Anderson.

Anderson's rise to fame is well documented. It started with one of those astronomically rare "getting discovered" moments. She was attending a BC Lions football game in Vancouver when her image was projected on the stadium's screen. The crowd cheered and, just like that, Anderson's career took off. She started in commercials, did the first of several *Playboy* spreads (she holds the record for the most *Playboy* covers at thirteen), and, soon after, landed a variety of TV roles, including the iconic part of swimsuit-wearing C. J. Parker on *Baywatch*.

Just how famous was (and *is*) Anderson? In 2005 she was named the top web-search term *ever*, ahead of "Christmas," "NFL," and "September 11." (Christmas needs a better publicist, obviously.) One online survey has her listed as the eighty-third most famous person in human history, behind Aristotle and Ernest Hemingway. She ranks well above that other ancient philosopher, Plato, on the fame gauge. And she also ranks high on numerous other best/most/sexiest lists. The music channel VH1's "Top 40 Hottest Hotties of the 90s"—yes, this is an official list—has her at number 2, just ahead of Brad Pitt and Cindy Crawford. I appreciate that inventories like the Hottest Hotties are hardly scientifically robust data, but they demonstrate the cultural space Anderson occupies.

Anderson's fame is also closely linked to cosmetic surgery. To put it bluntly: she has the world's most famous breast implants. No contest. No other celebrity even comes close. And there is at least some evidence that this reality is both a significant part of her celebrity status and, for better or worse, her most socially noteworthy and measurable contribution. In 2008 the International Society of Aesthetic Surgery surveyed more than twenty thousand plastic surgeons in eighty-four countries about the influence of celebrities on patients' choices. The society found that breasts and lips were the leading celebrity attributes desired by patients and that "the clear choice for breast look-alikes was Pamela Anderson." In addition, as sociologist Anthony Elliott reported in a 2011 article on the impact of celebrity culture, Anderson is one of the "key representatives of the celebrity-led plastic surgery revolution." Other scholars have noted that the rise and fall of Anderson's breast size—she has had several surgeries, including augmentations and subsequent reductions—reflects, and to some degree influences, broader social tastes associated with this particular part of human anatomy.

I have always been genuinely impressed by the way Anderson manages her public image. She projects a certain charm and unpretentious likability. And it was my impression that she has been able to maximize her famous-for-being-famous status by mixing in a dash of irony and perfectly calibrated self-deprecating humor. But, to my surprise, Anderson doesn't agree with me. In fact, she doesn't think she has an image that has been in any way manufactured or managed.

During the early stages of my research for this book, I had an odd e-mail exchange with Pamela Anderson. I had thought of her as an ideal person to engage on the topic of beauty and celebrity culture, particularly given her relationship to cosmetic surgery and the TV show *Baywatch*, which was more about breasts and bathing suits than plot and character. Though she initially was keen to do an interview, I got the sense that she did not like the direction taken by the questions I sent her, some of which asked about her exercise and beauty routine and others of which explored the tension between celebrity image and reality. She set the tone thus: "I may be the worst candidate for this line of questioning . . . I will be honest with you, if you are looking for the celebrity who worked hard to 'obtain a look,' keep looking." Later Anderson was more specific, stating: "I was and still am a Tom boy." And, in response to a question about whether she was aware that she was creating an iconic look: "No, just being myself—and I was working—I was playing Characters."

Perhaps she was toying with me. Perhaps she set the mode of her response to maximum tongue-in-cheek. I'll never know. But I think it only fair to take her responses at face value. And that leaves us with an intriguing paradox. The woman who has, one could forcefully argue, done more than almost any celebrity to facilitate the growth of an industry—cosmetic surgery—that is, at its core, about taking active and rather drastic steps to obtain a particular look, feels she has done little to shape her image. She also claimed an aversion to the concept of celebrity, a point she alluded to several times. She told me: "I really do not appreciate the word 'celebrity.' It's inhumane—and unattractive. I use my position in life to do as much as I can to help animals, the environment, the oceans, children."

YEARS AGO I HAD a brief encounter with Ms. Anderson. I was in the corner of an airport lounge, working and waiting for an international flight. Anderson and her small entourage sat immediately behind me. We exchanged a few words about something meaningless like the password to the wi-fi connection or the weather. She was pleasant and polite. She was wearing a form-fitting jumpsuit that was cut in a cleavage-friendly manner. I remember thinking, "Gosh, she is a tiny person" and "Where does one buy a form-fitting, low-cut jumpsuit?" But at no point did I think, "Now here sits a tomboy."

AS MY EXCHANGES with Anderson underscore, the relationship of celebrities, body image, and the actions we take to modify our looks is ridiculously convoluted. Anderson's career, no doubt, benefited hugely from her unique image, and that image is closely associated with cosmetic surgery, even if she sees it differently. No matter what she says or thinks, her cultural impact has been significant. The image of Anderson has a life of its own. And it can pull off a form-fitting jumpsuit.

IT IS IMPORTANT to acknowledge, if only briefly, that the influence of celebrity culture on our perceptions of beauty is not always, or necessarily, negative. Celebrity status can also be used, for example, to break stereotypes and reframe the relationship of sexuality, gender, and social roles. Some celebrities, such as Lady Gaga, have explicitly stated that they have a feminist agenda (admittedly, not everyone buys the claim). Other celebrities, such as the actor Olivia Munn, view fame as an opportunity to chip away at the female caricatures so dominant in popular culture. Munn, a comedian (she was a faux, and hilarious, correspondent on *The Daily Show*) and a TV and movie star (e.g., *Magic Mike*, *Ironman 2*, and HBO's *The Newsroom*), has been criticized in some circles for her willingness to appear in mainstream media, such as the cover of the men's magazine *Maxim*. This and similar career decisions have certainly raised her profile, resulting, for example, in frequent appearances on those ubiquitous annual "sexiest women" lists. Munn argues that these criticisms flow from a double standard. "There's apparently no way that I can embrace my sexuality, be on the cover of a men's magazine, and also be thoughtful and smart, and know what the Pythagorean theorem is," she says.

I asked Munn, undoubtedly a rising star, what she views as the biggest perk of fame. I expected her to tell me something about how well she is now treated or that she loves working with terrific actors and directors. I got a much different response. "The best thing about fame is that it can be used to break down barriers," she says. "The entertainment business perpetuates stereotypes—from movies and TV to billboards and magazine covers—and it's nice when you're in a position to help perpetuate a different stereotype, one that hopefully helps change perceptions, even if it's in a very small way." This response, no doubt, is aimed at her critics.

A number of academics I interviewed hold a view similar to Munn's. They note that celebrities can use their status to (I hesitate to use this word, but here I go) empower women and give them agency over their body and sexuality. In addition, taking ownership of an image or stereotype can change its cultural meaning (think of the evolution of "the blonde" from Marilyn Monroe to Madonna). I won't dive too deeply into this debate. But I will say that there is, no doubt, a delicate balance between producing images that may promote empowerment and those that are simply aesthetically pleasing and, as such, play to existing stereotypes. The average guy probably doesn't care about Lady Gaga's intention when she wears next to nothing. I simply want to highlight that this is a complex part of the story.

Pornification

"It used to be all about boobs, now it is all about the ass," Vanessa tells me. Her close friend and former coworker, Elena, nods in agreement. The two women—petite, curvy, and quick to smile—should know. They are both adult entertainment actors or, as the rest of the world usually describes their vocation, porn stars. Vanessa's San Fernando Valley apartment is spacious and tastefully furnished. She is an aspiring artist, and her striking work hangs on the wall behind the sofa. The paintings are big, graphic, and sexual. They feature naked women on their backs with their legs open, eyes locked on some unknown observer.

"I took the images from an old *Penthouse* magazine and tried to interpret them in a more beautiful and playful manner," Vanessa tells me. I immediately think of obvious metaphors for her life but say nothing. Vanessa, who studied art in New York before her porn career, is returning to painting because the porn industry is dying, even here in the Valley, a locale that has long been the center of the US industry. This is happening for numerous reasons, but the biggest factor is the availability of free Internet porn. If people don't need to pay, they won't.

Another challenge: there are more and more "porn girls," as they are called in the industry, willing to do just about anything for less and less money. This flood of eager actors is partly the result of the main-streaming of porn and the belief that it will be a portal to conventional, Hollywood-style, celebrity. One of the few studies on point, published in 2013, found that a desire for money and fame are the two most common reasons people get into the porn industry.

"Many girls, young girls, get into porn because they think they are going to be famous," Vanessa says.

"It is true," Elena says. "Some new girls think they *are* famous just because they have had sex on camera a few times." Both actors punctuate this last comment with eye rolls and under-their-breath expletives.

"How young?" I ask.

"Eighteen," they respond in unison.

For Vanessa, the porn industry has, in the relatively recent past, been quite lucrative. She often made more than the industry standard of $1,000 per sex act (pay depends, in part, on the nature of the activity). And it has, indeed, been a ticket into the world of Hollywood's rich and famous. She is a friend—in some cases, a good friend—of many A-list celebrities. (She asks me not to name names, but it did not take much Googling to confirm the connections.) She tells me matter-of-factly about wild parties at which guests are required to deposit their cell phones before they enter. "You'd be surprised how many celebrities like to hang with porn stars," she says. I mention a big-name movie star who has a stellar reputation as a family man. "Him too," she says. "Many of my friends have partied at his house." (I am not sure if *partied* is a euphemism for a broad range of party-like activities. I don't ask. My lack of journalistic tenacity will later irritate many curious friends and family.)

Given this kind of glamour—or, at least, the proximity to glamour—you can, I suppose, understand the allure of the porn star's profession. And, I admit, just hearing about it prompts a certain thrill. Many of us, perhaps most, are fascinated by the party habits of celebrities, especially if they involve a throng of porn stars. And if Vanessa's and Elena's descriptions are even half accurate, it sounds as though clothes are often optional and that, for some odd reason, much of the partying happens in kitchens and ridiculously opulent bathrooms. But it should not be forgotten that reaching even Vanessa's level of renown is vanishingly rare, especially as porn's profitability diminishes. Indeed, an odd paradox is unfolding in popular culture. Porn has, arguably, never had more social salience—as witnessed by the porn star–inspired style choices ("porn chic," as it is often called) of celebs such as Miley Cyrus and Rihanna. And porn has never been more mainstream. Explicit porn to satisfy almost any taste can be accessed—and, if you believe the research on point, *is* being accessed—at any moment on a computer or smartphone. As a result, porn now appears to be a less extreme career choice than it once was. This is happening at a time when achieving fame through porn is becoming less and less likely. (I will refrain from commenting on the personal costs often associated with this career choice, including ubiquitous drug use and the exploitation of naive newbies who don't know what they've signed up for—two issues noted by both Vanessa and Elena.) In other words, the same forces—mostly, free Internet porn—that are normalizing porn and making it seem like a vehicle to fame are also making the likelihood of generating fame by way of a successful porn career less and less probable.

"There just isn't as much work," Vanessa says. "And there aren't as many porn blockbusters making girls well known."

Of course, porn is also having a profound influence on more than just the fashion choices of pop stars and the career ambitions of celebrity wannabes. The current pornsplosion, as some commentators have called it, is also having a measurable impact on notions of beauty and what is deemed erotic, as illustrated by Vanessa and Elena's observation regarding the shift in focus from the bosom to the derriere. And, at the same time, porn is having an effect on the popularity of a range of cosmetic services, including nipple tattooing (the darkening and reshaping of the areola), anal bleaching (the lightening of the area around . . . well, you get the idea), and, most significantly, cosmetic genital surgery.

Over the past few years there has been a huge increase in the number of procedures aimed at producing an aesthetically pleasing vagina. We live in the era of the designer vagina. Currently, thousands of these procedures are performed each year, and its popularity is growing. In the US the number of cosmetic vagina procedures is up 64 percent since 2011. A

2013 study by a UK industry group reported a similar rise. It also found that the average age of patients has dropped significantly in recent years, from thirty-five to twenty-eight.

As with all forms of cosmetic surgery, the reasons patients seek it out are varied and complex. Some women who get this procedure may have profound labial asymmetry or a functional impairment. But it seems difficult to deny that both the growth in the practice and the particular aesthetic that is now popular—a prepubescent look that includes small labia and a flattened vulva—are a direct result of porn. A recent study published in the *International Journal of Gynecology and Obstetrics* lends support to this speculation. The study found that women who viewed images of women with surgically altered vulvas were more likely than a control group to view modified genitalia as normal, and, the authors speculate, this helps to explain why healthy women seek genital surgery.

Dr. Jennifer Blake, the chief executive officer of the Society of Obstetricians and Gynaecologists of Canada (SOGC) and a respected gynecologist, told me that she too believes the popularity of the procedure is a direct result of the easy access to porn. Indeed, she doesn't know how else the phenomenon could have emerged. "Of course, the fashion is now little or no hair down there," she tells me. "This makes everything more visible and has added to the pressure to change how you look. But porn is a big factor." And she feels strongly that the preference for a flat and child-like vulva, which, as an article in the *British Journal of General Practice* noted is a recent trend, is likely to be transient. "Who knows what will be popular and viewed as erotic in the future? The aesthetic is going to change," Blake says. And that is a problem because this is a very permanent alteration. "What's gone is gone. If a problem emerges or you change your mind, you can't go back," Blake tells me.

The irreversibility of genital surgery could be problematic for a number of reasons. Many doctors worry about potential health risks. "There is absolutely no long-term data. Zero," Blake notes emphatically. The UK Royal College of Obstetricians and Gynaecologists echoed her concern when it noted that the amount of tissue removed is comparable to forms of genital mutilation, a practice associated with a number of serious, long-term complications. In fact, a 2012 article published in *Obstetrician & Gynaecologist* suggested that there "is limited evidence to allow women to give informed consent."

A 2012 study published in the *British Medical Journal* looked at how clinics advertise this procedure. It was found that they often promise a "'youthful' vulval appearance" or labia that are "'sleeker' and 'more appealing'" or that the procedure will allow you to "'feel like a real woman again.'" The study concluded that "unsubstantiated claims of physical, psychological and sexual benefits were present on every website."

Some legal and ethics scholars have argued that female genital cosmetic surgery, unless done for the health of the patient, should be illegal, because it exploits vulnerable women and, like female genital mutilation done for cultural and religious reasons, has many risks. Two Oxford University academics have argued that female genital cosmetic surgery is *already* illegal in England under the terms of the Female Genital Mutilation Act, which states that it is a criminal offense "for a person to excise, infibulate, or otherwise mutilate any part of a girl's labia minora, majora or clitoris." In other countries, such as Canada, it is also a criminal offense, unless the woman is older than eighteen (which is the norm in the context of cosmetic procedures) or if the procedure is done by a medical professional in order to benefit the physical health of the woman or, according to the criminal code, to ensure she has "normal reproductive functions or normal sexual appearance." Of course, there are many significant differences between female genital mutilation—often inflicted on young women without their consent and in less than ideal clinical circumstances—and female genital cosmetic surgery performed with her consent and by regulated professionals. Still, similarities do exist—comparable procedures, cultural pressures that shape notions of normality, and unknown risks—between a universally condemned act and one that is growing in popularity and acceptance. This highlights the power of celebrity culture to influence social norms and motivate and normalize relatively extreme acts.

# # #

BEFORE LEAVING VANESSA'S APARTMENT, I ask her about the phenomenon of the perfect vagina in the context of the porn industry. What is the
expectation? Given her look of befuddlement, I assume this was a stupid
question with an obvious answer. "If you don't have a nice pussy, you
shouldn't be in porn," she says.

Is It Worth It?

One of the primary reasons that people get cosmetic surgery, particularly
alterations to the face, is to look younger and more attractive. Yes, as I
have already noted, the motivations are complex and multiple. And I
don't mean to imply that getting cosmetic surgery is always a mistake.
Still, few could argue with the proposition that rejuvenation and beauty
enhancement are core motivations and central to the marketing of the
industry. But, it turns out that, despite the dramatic nature of such procedures, cosmetic surgery's impact in both these respects can in fact be
relatively modest.

A 2013 study published in the *JAMA Facial Plastic Surgery* sought to
assess the degree to which cosmetic surgery—including face-lifts, brow
lifts, and eyelid surgery—made people look younger and more attractive.
The researchers had people rate the age and attractiveness of patients before and after surgery. The raters didn't know if they were looking at a
before or after image. It turned out that the cosmetic surgery decreased
the perception of age by a modest 3.1 years and, more shockingly, had almost *no* impact on attractiveness. Other research using similar methods,
such as a 2011 study on the rejuvenating effects of rhinoplasty (nose jobs),
had similarly modest results.

This surprising lack of impact has been found using other approaches.
For example, another study, published in 2012, looked at the value of
beautification from an economic perspective. The authors, Soohyung Lee
and Keunkwan Ryu, were curious to learn whether cosmetic surgery was
worth it, money wise. Beautiful people do make more money than their
less aesthetically blessed peers, but would the costs of cosmetic surgery
be offset by an increase in income? The results are consistent with the

data from the other studies I've discussed. The study found, in general, that "the improvement in beauty due to plastic surgery is small." And, as a result, the beauty "benefit is, on average, not large enough to justify the surgery costs." In reaching the latter conclusion, Lee and Ryu considered increases in income from both employment and marriage. It is worth noting that a 2002 study—led by the well-known economist Daniel Hamermesh—came to a similar conclusion regarding spending on cosmetics and clothing. The researchers found that the impact on beauty of even a large amount of money was not huge. Most women will make back only about 15 percent of their investment in clothes and cosmetics from a beauty-boosted bump in income.

To be fair, some studies, including a 2012 analysis from Canada, found that cosmetic surgery could reduce the perception of age, particularly if a number of procedures were done. And surgery that corrects disfigurements or congenital abnormalities can have a dramatic impact. But, in general, the data on the impact of cosmetic surgery to combat aging and enhance beauty is underwhelming. In other words, if looking younger and more attractive is your motivation for cosmetic surgery, keep your expectations low. As the Royal College of Surgeons noted in its 2013 report, no one can or should promise nicer or better, just different.

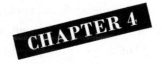

Wired Behavior

So far I've tried to show how most beautifying activities either do not work or achieve much less than advertised. So you won't be surprised to learn that my general advice is to ignore all these products and procedures. Save your money and spare yourself the psychic angst. And I stand by that conclusion.

But here is the crushing and seemingly contradictory truth: despite all my musings about the futility of most beautification activities, no one can deny that beauty really does matter. It matters a lot. Sure, it may be only skin deep, but the picture that skin provides to the universe has real social, economic, and romantic consequences. Indeed, it matters on so many levels that it is difficult to find a realm of social interaction where looks don't have at least some impact, usually, but not always, conferring a significant benefit on those lucky enough to be beautiful. I wish the data painted a different picture. I wish I could say that the beautiful enjoy no long-term benefit. I wish I could say that we all look past appearance and measure other humans solely on such traits as character, sincerity, kindness, and wit. It seems deeply unfair. But, like it or not, we are wired to be superficial.

This reality is hardly news. I think most of us know that looks are important. And despite a few decades' worth of academic pontification that our reverence for beauty is a social construct created by a largely male-dominated world, few in the academic community now doubt the social power and enduring nature of our love affair with good looks. "I sort out what it means," Daniel Hamermesh told me. "I measure its impact. Whether it is the result of genetics, evolution, or how we are raised, I don't think about that stuff, but I know beauty has an impact. The research is completely unequivocal."

The power and influence of beauty appear to be the result of a complex combination of evolutionarily determined, hardwired biological preferences and socially constructed taste. Whether nature or nurture is decisive is moot. Some of the academics I spoke to leaned toward the former explanation, others toward the latter. I have no intention of siding with one or the other, as I think it is so obviously a blend of both. What folks in medieval rural England viewed as sexy and hot—perhaps a full set of reasonably healthy teeth—is obviously not what is considered sexy and hot in Hollywood today. Taste evolves and is not, in general, universal. While almost all researchers agree that at least some of what we find attractive (in women this means smooth skin, symmetrical features, and an hourglass figure; in men, it means being tall and having a variety of other attributes I lack) is evolutionarily imprinted on our brains, there is abundant evidence that the local environment, whether a post-Pleistocene African savannah or a pop culture–saturated suburb, can have a tangible effect on those preferences.

A fascinating study published in 2013 in the journal *Human Nature* demonstrated the degree to which our taste in mates is the result of a complex and ever-changing nature-nurture mashup. A previous line of research found that most men find women with relatively small feet to be more attractive than women with large feet. If there are two women who are identical except for the size of their feet, men will, on average, pick the woman with the smaller feet. An individual with a foot fetish could probably provide a more nuanced explanation for this phenomenon, but for the purpose of this study, size was the sole (no pun intended) variable. However, the 2013 study found that admiration for little feet is not universal. The author, anthropologist Geoff Kushnick, found that approximately 150 adult male members of Karo Batak, a relatively isolated agricultural community in rural Indonesia, had a "marked pref-erence for women with large feet." When the results from Indonesia were compared with the preferences of men from all over the world, Kushnick concluded that exposure to Western culture was correlated with a preference for small feet and that preference for big feet was likely adaptive. "In the Karo Batak communities I studied," Kushnick noted, "men were overheard saying that a woman with larger feet was stronger and thus more productive in the rice fields." This study nicely highlights that even a seemingly universal and allegedly biologically determined preference can be influenced by local conditions and that the popular culture influences those preferences. Apparently, the more you see small feet in magazines and movies and on TV, the less sexy those big, strong, productive feet look.

Numerous other studies remind us of the biological and unconscious foundations of our preferences. There is little doubt, for instance, that traits that signal a woman's health and fertility are attractive to men. One interesting study (and a depressing one, if you are an anxiety-ridden and overworked woman) from 2013, undertaken at the University of Turku in Finland, found that stress makes women's faces less attractive to men. Specifically, the researchers found that the cortisol levels in the blood (a marker for stress) are significantly and independently associated with the perceived attractiveness of a woman's face. The authors speculate that indications of stress serve as a signal of "both how healthy someone is as well as their fertility." This is, no doubt, evolution at work. Men aren't thinking, *Wow, look at those low cortisol levels . . . that is seriously sexy!* For most of human history, finding a mate who was not under a lot of stress—meaning that he or she had access to food, wasn't under constant threat of being eaten by a lion, and so on—was a good thing. It presumed a greater chance of passing on your genes.

Another physical trait that we all find attractive, particularly in women, is even skin tone. Again, this likely relates to evolutionarily de-termined tastes. A study published in 2010, for example, found that men could detect even a small change in skin surface topography and that it had a direct impact on judgments of attractiveness. Another study tracked the gaze (and number of "fixations") of men as they looked at pictures of female faces. The authors found that variation of skin tone was an independent predictor of attractiveness. The more homogeneous the skin, the better. This characteristic is, of course, also a visual cue for health, fertility, and, most of all, youth.

So what does the research tell us? Hamermesh, one of the leading authorities on the economics of beauty, conducted one of the first studies, now considered a classic, on the social value of beauty. He remembers well the date the results of his groundbreaking study were first released, because Jay Leno used it as the basis for a joke in his monologue. It was 1993 and the joke was so 1993. It went something like this: If attractive people earn more money, then why does Ross Perot earn more than Rob Lowe?

Despite Leno's skepticism, Hamermesh's data are pretty convincing. Attractive people make more money. Period. Worse, people with below-average looks are penalized more than the attractive are rewarded. Hamermesh and his coauthor, Jeff Biddle, found that attractive people earn, on average, a premium of about 5 percent and homely people—as the authors bluntly categorize this cohort—are penalized by about 9 percent. These were confirmed in a 2009 study that found a similar "plainness penalty" of 3 to 5 percent. The researchers also found that for attractive individuals, an increase in skill and ability is associated with an even greater increase in wages, while added ability in those who have below-average looks may lead to *less* pay! Harsh.

Since the publication of his seminal paper, Hamermesh's work has been confirmed and refined again and again. For example, a 2006 paper found the existence of a beauty premium (this paper suggests that good-looking people earn about 10 to 15 percent more than their homelier counterparts) and broke down its source. The authors found that some of the beauty premium is likely the result of such factors as the greater confidence that attractive people usually possess, but the major factor is looks. Another study takes the we-are-a-bunch-of-superficial-animals theme even further by highlighting the economic benefits of being blonde. Using data from more than twelve thousand American women, the authors found that blondes receive a significant wage premium—equivalent to about an extra year of postsecondary education! Moreover, they marry men who make about 6 percent more than the husbands of women who lack the flaxen advantage. Blondes may not have more fun, but they have a bit of extra cash to pay for fun stuff.

The social advantages conferred on the gorgeous go well beyond making more money. A fascinating 2013 study, again led by Hamermesh, found that the good-looking are significantly happier and more satisfied than the plain. The large study, which includes data from all over the world, found that beauty increases happiness both directly (*Golly, it sure is terrific being attractive!*) and indirectly, as a result of such factors as greater earning power and a better education.

One of my favorite studies observed that people do not, at least when they are contestants on TV game shows and under the watchful eye of the public audience, discriminate on the basis of race or gender. But, holy cow, they sure do discriminate on the basis of looks! The 2012 study found that good-looking people are less likely to be eliminated from a show, even if they perform more poorly than their average-looking fellow contestants. The authors note that this phenomenon is simply a form of taste-based discrimination and, given that contestant decisions are scrutinized by the public, stands as strong evidence of how acceptable and insidious the beauty premium is.

And it doesn't stop there. Attractive people are regarded as more moral. Good-looking students get better grades. And beautiful people even have better, more adventurous sex. In fact, women are more likely to have an orgasm if their partner is handsome and, in particular, symmetrical . . . in the face, that is.

The beauty advantage has been confirmed using a wide range of methods. For example, a 2011 study by neuroscientists at Duke University found that our brains have a shared neural pathway for the assessment of goodness and beauty. This provides biological support for the beauty-is-good stereotype (i.e., the tendency to believe good-looking individuals are more moral, etc.). This notion is, to some degree, hardwired. Specifically, the researchers found "a positive bias toward attractiveness and goodness coupled with a negative bias against unattractiveness and badness." Research also suggests this bias is quite difficult to overcome, even if you are aware of it. A 2014 study out of the University of Toronto found that first impressions about an individual—which are based largely on appearance—are hard to alter. As one of the authors put it: "We judge books by their covers, and we can't help but do it," and "first impressions continue to assert themselves long after you know relevant information about a person." I could go on but you get the idea. Beauty matters.

Given this reality, it should be no surprise that those who are deemed unattractive pay a heavy social price and not just in terms of financial compensation. A 2013 study, for example, found that unattractive individuals are significantly more likely to be abused at work. While many studies show that good-looking kids get treated better than homely kids, this is one of the first studies to find a link between looks and workplace behavior. Sadly, looks-mediated bullying persists into adulthood. As noted by the authors, the reasons are simple: "Attractive people may be aesthetically pleasant to others, eliciting positive emotion, while unattractive people may be aesthetically unpleasant to others, eliciting negative emotion." Unattractive people have also been found to have an increased propensity toward criminal behavior, even when you control for other relevant factors, such as socioeconomic status. And, to add insult to injury, the same line of research has found that attractive people have a *reduced* propensity toward crime.

There are a few downsides to being good-looking. For example, if you find yourself convicted of murder and you are also kind of hot, you are more likely to be presumed guilty. So, before you hit the courtroom, ugly yourself up a bit. (Perhaps this explains why the pre-arrest style of boyfriend-killer Jodi Arias was classic blonde bombshell and her in-court vibe leaned more toward dowdy librarian.) Also, while good-looking men are more employable than their plain-looking colleagues, there is some evidence that attractive women don't have the same advantage—at least in the initial callback phase of the hiring process. One study found that attractive women who included a picture with their resume were significantly less likely to get an interview than women who either sent no picture or whose picture showed them to be plain-looking. The authors of the study conclude: "Female jealousy of attractive women in the workplace is a primary reason for the punishment of attractive women." Ouch.

Given our established obsession with beauty—driven, in part, by celebrity culture, a point I'll return to—you won't be surprised to learn that, despite society's efforts to fight discrimination, the effect of the beauty premium does not seem to be fading. A recent Australian study by Jeff Borland and Andrew Leigh found that since the mid-1980s the premium conferred on the good-looking has been constant and, in fact, has increased slightly for females as assessed by the likelihood of their being employed. While Hamermesh finds it gratifying that his early work continues to be confirmed, he is genuinely disappointed by the resilience of the beauty premium. "Why in God's name does it still exist? Ugly people can be just as smart and can reproduce just as well!" he told me. "This is a powerful force. As a source of discrimination [the economic data tell us], that is not that much different from race." As Nancy Etcoff notes in her seminal book on this point, *Survival of the Prettiest*, "We face a world where 'lookism' is one of the most pervasive but denied of prejudices." To be fair, there have been a few recent legal actions challenging lookism. A protest group made a big public relations splash in 2013 and threatened legal action if the retail giant Abercrombie & Fitch continued to employ only good-looking people in its flagship store in Paris. But, in general, our socially and biologically driven preference for attractive people is wholly unchecked. Beauty rules.

The Clock Is Ticking

Our society is obsessed with youth. And many researchers have suggested that this obsession has an evolutionary foundation. We don't want to age, at least not in appearance, and we find youthfulness sexy. Celebrity culture amplifies and reflects this obsession, as does the entire beauty and antiaging industry—an industry that is growing rapidly as the average age of the world population nudges upward. I think this cultural fixation is obvious and axiomatic. I don't need to convince anyone of its existence,

but I will say this: in the world of Hollywood image makers, the obsession borders on insanity, particularly for women.

"I know the value of my work is more than my looks. It is confusing
for me that I must look a certain way, but the industry expects that. It
is . . . [long pause] confusing." Kyla Wise said that last word through a
half-smile, followed by a sigh and shoulder slump. We met at a coffee
shop to talk about the challenges of being an actor, but it quickly became
a discussion about the challenges of being a *female* actor.

Wise, who made her television debut as Sapphire on *Honey, I Shrunk
the Kids: The TV Show*, in 1997, is so unmistakably attractive that it
seems absurd that the issue would concern her. But such is the entertainment industry. Just so there is no confusion, Wise is the kind of attractive that causes strangers—mostly men, naturally—to pretend they
are not staring. I assume they are thinking, "Why is *that* woman sitting
with *that* doofus?"

She has already had a solid acting career, which started immediately
after she graduated from university with a bachelor of fine arts in drama.
She is no lightweight. She won the department's gold medal. Since then
she has had guest and recurring roles on numerous TV shows. And she
has been in both independent and Hollywood movies. The work has
been steady. Still, despite the enviable resume, it is no surprise that Wise
is now both philosophical and apprehensive about her future. She is turn-
ing forty—the big 4-0—two days after our interview. I caught her on the
cusp of a big threshold, so the issues of looks and age have been weighing
on her. And who can blame her? She is, after all, a female actor.

"Once [women] hit thirty, things get tough. In fact, there are few
parts for women past thirty-five. There are character roles, but not many,"
T. W. Peacocke tells me. He is an award-winning Canadian film and TV
director, so this is a trend he has witnessed firsthand. "The classic example
is the movie *North by Northwest*. Cary Grant's mother is played by Jessie
Royce Landis, and she is only a few years [eight, actually] older than
Grant. For women, there really is a ticking clock."

Peacocke's comments may seem harsh and cynical. But, sadly, mountains of cruel data support his observations. The writer Kyle Buchanan,

for example, recently published an article in which he compared the age of ten leading men and the ages of the actors cast as their romantic interests. He looked at nine to eleven movies for each of the stars. The results were unambiguous. First, the age gap in a number of cases was ridiculous. Consider, for example, Steve Carell (forty-nine) and Keira Knightley (twenty-seven) in *Seeking a Friend for the End of the World*, Liam Neeson (sixty-one) and Olivia Wilde (twenty-nine) in *Third Person*, and Johnny Depp (forty-eight) and Amber Heard (twenty-five) in *The Rum Diary*. More disturbing is that, for women, hitting age forty really does seem to be a major obstacle or, more accurately, a career cliff over which they tumble and disappear. Of the 102 movies Buchanan considered, only eighteen had a romantic female lead over forty, and in most of those movies the male lead was substantially older, with only a handful of exceptions (for example, Richard Gere, fifty-five, and Susan Sarandon, fifty-eight, in *Shall We Dance*). Indeed, about 70 percent of the female leads were thirty-five or younger. The message is clear: men can get older, but women must remain the same age.

Many academic studies confirm this enduring age and gender bias. A 2002 study of the one hundred highest-grossing films found that the majority of female actors were in their twenties and thirties, while the majority of males were in their thirties and forties. Another comprehensive study, of films released between 1926 and 1999, traced the negative effect that getting on in years has on a woman's acting career. The authors of the study concluded "that men are allowed to age in film, and women are not. Male stars in their sixties are routinely cast as leads, even in physically demanding roles. Conversely, female stars are rarely cast as leads after they enter their forties."

Almost every corner of popular culture shares this age bias, but none more so than the fashion industry. Ashley Mears is uniquely qualified to comment on this reality—she has explored the fashion industry from the inside (she has modeled for such designers as Marc Jacobs) and is now a professor of sociology at Boston University. Mears, whose research has found that modeling is a pretty brutal and surprisingly low-paying job (a point I will return to), tells me that "many models are recruited as

young as thirteen and the average age for a high-fashion model is probably twenty-three or twenty-four, but many are as young as seventeen."
While Mears thinks there has been a healthy "growth in the critique and
in the public awareness of this situation," she also feels that it will be hard
to remedy because, as she notes, "young and thin still sells." She thinks
change will have to come from the outside, that we need laws to nudge
the entire fashion industry toward a more realistic portrayal of women.

It is no surprise, then, that study after study supports the tight connection between youth and beauty. A 2012 study, to cite just one example,
found that attractive faces strike us as looking young, and we consider
young faces to be more attractive. Given this reality, who could blame
celebrities and the general public for scrambling to avoid a damaged der-
mis? A 2013 UK survey of more than two thousand women found that 91
percent were worried about the effects of aging on their appearance and a
remarkable 75 percent said they were already using some kind of product
to fight those effects. And women aren't the only ones who are worried.
Men are an increasingly large part of the market for antiaging products.
A survey of more than a thousand men revealed that approximately 60
percent of men between eighteen and thirty-four regularly buy beauty
products for their skin but tend to keep it a secret. The purveyors of
antiaging products, meanwhile, have helped to make aging seem almost
unnatural, as if it is an ailment. A 2012 study of 124 advertisements for
antiaging products found several key and consistent themes, including
the use of scientific language to make the products seem like a drug that
could cure the disease of aging and, as the author put it, a twisted logic
that equated youth with beauty and femininity and "older age with the
absence of these qualities." The study found that the expectation that we
should try to remain youthful, no matter what it takes, has been made
to seem normal.

KYLA WISE IS A POSITIVE PERSON. She loves acting and wants her career to
continue. She wants it to thrive. She tells me that she continues to take
classes and to audition for good parts, and she has started teaching. And,

by the way, she could easily pass for twenty-nine. But she is frustrated. "I constantly ask myself, How do I stay competitive in a competitive business when they expect youth and a certain look? There are lots of mixed messages," Wise says. Mixed messages? I don't think so. The message is uniform, oppressively consistent, and crystal clear. Don't age.

Celebrity Comparisons

If you are a man and you lived in a world where Homer Simpson was your primary point of comparison, chances are you would feel pretty good about yourself. If you saw only Homeresque people strolling the streets and pictured in magazines, on TV, and in movies—both from Hollywood and of the . . . er, homemade, erotic variety—than you would probably feel that you stacked up well against the rest of the universe. While you might feel compelled to stay fit and eat well for health purposes and psychological well-being, aesthetic competition probably wouldn't be a big motivator. In a beauty competition—and we all seem to be in one big, never-ending pageant, where we are all simultaneously judges and competitors—you'd likely perform pretty well. (Sorry, Homer.) But we men don't live in Homerworld. We live in a world saturated with images of Brad Pitt, Johnny Depp, Channing Tatum, Justin Timberlake, Tom Brady, and that damn Daniel Craig (my wife's favorite). These are our comparators. Against these guys, most of us do not do so well.

For women, of course, the situation is much, much worse. It is worse in every way imaginable. Popular culture is completely drenched in images of young, thin women. In many ways, the dominant image of modern popular culture *is* young, thin women. They may not always be in the frame, but they are never far from view. One study, for example, found that 94 percent of the female characters on TV are thinner than the average woman. Ninety-eight percent of professional models are skinnier than average (no surprise) and have a BMI (somewhere between 15 and 17) that places them in the category of unhealthily underweight. And, as I have noted, older women are largely erased from, or marginalized in, almost all forms of popular culture. At least Brad and Johnny are about my age. For women, the pop-culture comparator is almost always a female who looks like a teenager or a woman who just left her teenage years. (Gwyneth helps: she is older than forty!) A Canadian study, published in 2011, determined that the idealized images of women portrayed in magazines and on TV are much more homogeneous and rigid (again, extremely young and thin) than media images of men.

While much research still needs to be done on the interplay of celebs and how we view our own physical attractiveness, one area that has received a great deal of attention is a phenomenon called "social comparison." The concept is simple: We are neurologically wired and socialized to measure ourselves against other humans, whether we know it or not. We rank our success, looks, and status against others'. Brain-imaging research, including a 2013 study done by researchers from Germany and the United Kingdom, has reinforced the idea that this phenomenon has a biological underpinning. Specifically, the German-UK team explored how the brain weighs "someone's attractiveness in relation to a given standard." It turns out that our brains treat beauty in the same way as other, more objectively quantifiable traits such as height. We simply contrast one person's looks (even our own, I suspect) against the comparator's. Indeed, we compare beauty with the same part of the brain that we use to compare height, which suggests that social comparison is hardwired even for something as socially mediated and seemingly subjective as beauty.

In general, we compare upward, particularly in the arena of looks. (As I will discuss, we also frequently compare downward, perhaps to someone we believe to be less attractive—often to make ourselves feel better!) Upward comparison can be inspiring, but research shows that it can also be disheartening, particularly for those who have preexisting issues with body image. Indeed, study after study has suggested that by creating an idealized standard of beauty—one that leaves us *all*, to a greater or lesser degree, wanting—celebrity culture helps to generate a social norm that is far from constructive and, I have no doubt, helps to drive the beauty industry.

Studies consistently show that media images can have an adverse (though perhaps short-term) impact on our mood and satisfaction with respect to our appearance and weight. A 2010 study of more than one hundred women found that viewing idealized images of women (e.g., fashion models and celebrities) caused a social comparison that had a negative impact on mood. Another study, published in 2013, explored the impact of media on women who were trying to eat less (which, these days, is about 25 percent of the adult population) and came to a similar conclusion, that "restrained eaters exposed to media images reported decreased weight satisfaction and increased negative mood." This kind of conclusion is typical of the research in this area. And the tendency to compare upward to an idealized image seems particularly common for women. Numerous studies have found that women are more likely than men to make an upward comparison to an idealized and unrealistic norm.

While much of the existing research has focused on women, some studies suggest popular culture may have an impact on men and teenage boys too—though the effect is less pronounced. For example, a 2013 study found that adolescent boys who watched music videos containing muscular and attractive singers—I am guessing they didn't subject them to any Nickelback—"had poorer body satisfaction and poorer mood compared to boys who viewed average-looking singers."

So comparing ourselves to hot celebrities seems to have an impact on how we think about beauty and our own appearance, a phenomenon I have already described in the context of cosmetic surgery. And since we do not reside in Homerworld but in a celebrity-dominated universe, opportunities to make this comparison exist all day, every day.

How Hot Is Your Partner? Alas, Not Very

Before I move on, it is worth noting an obvious corollary to this social comparison stuff: idealized images of celebrities also affect how people rank the beauty of others. This is at least partly because of a psychological phenomenon called the contrast effect. A classic study published in 1980 found that men rank the attractiveness and dating desirability of a woman much lower after viewing media images of attractive females. Groups of men watched the TV show *Charlie's Angels* or looked at magazine ads containing beautiful women. (Yes, in 1980, the Angels, including the underappreciated Farrah Fawcett replacement, Tanya Roberts, helped set the standard for beauty.) This exposure had the predicted effect: women in the real world looked much less desirable.

Of course, given that we live in a world where images of idealized men and women are even more ubiquitous than in 1980—*Charlie's Angels* seems quaint in comparison to, say, the flesh on display in HBO's *Spartacus*, *True Blood*, or *Game of Thrones*—this contrast effect is likely operating at all times, skewing how men and women perceive the attractiveness of the "average" people we see all day long. This includes how you rate your current partner. A well-known study found that men who were asked to look at *Playboy*-type images of nude women subsequently rated their spouses as less attractive than if the comparison wasn't made.

Popular culture operates like a cruel, constantly operating dissatisfaction machine.

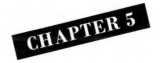

Beauty and/or Health?

Apparently, Christina Aguilera needed time off in 2013 from her hit TV show, *The Voice*, "to focus on herself," at least according to my go-to bedtime reading, *People*.

I am about six months into my routine as a *People* devotee, and I feel as if I have read hundreds of articles about celebrity weight loss. (In fact, 66 percent of the issues I read contained at least one article about weight loss or dieting, several of them featured on the cover.) They are almost always framed as admiring, good-for-her, inspirational tales. (And, yes, most featured female celebrities.) But this one about Aguilera stands out from the horde. First, the story has a striking presentation. The piece is built around multiple shots of Aguilera that highlight her weight during each phase of her career. It is, I think, meant to resemble that classic image of humans evolving in stages from a small, hunched, hairy ape to an upright, posture-improved human. The point, as captured in the headline "Body Evolution," is that Aguilera's body has evolved from curvy to sleek.

And this leads me to the second reason this article grabbed my attention: there is a cutting duplicity in the message. One of the largest photos, taken in 2012, is an image of Aguilera at her, well, largest. Under the photo is a quote from Aguilera from the day the photo was taken. "I embrace my body," said the then-full-figured singer. This line conveys an acceptance that humans come in all shapes and sizes. And, I am sure, that was the theme of the article when that quote was first published. But the point of the current piece is clearly that thin is best. It is a celebration of Aguilera's evolution to thinness—which, according to *People*, is the result of a "fresh start"—new boyfriend, new house, revamped lifestyle, and so on. As one of Aguilera's friends is quoted as saying, "She is shedding the past and shedding the pounds." Evidently, "focus on herself" is a celebrity-magazine euphemism for "lose lots of weight."

The idea that we all should be constantly evolving and improving—and that improving is equated almost entirely with aesthetic goals, such as weight loss, better skin, bigger boobs, perkier nose, more muscles, and the like—was a theme I came across again and again in the course of my research. "Seventy to 90 percent of women want to be thinner, and something like 60 percent of men want to be more muscular," Viren Swami, a professor in the Department of Psychology at the University of Westminster, told me as we sat in his London faculty office. "If you aren't working on your appearance, you aren't normal. If you opt out [of this cultural norm], you are derided and marginalized."

THERE ARE REASONS to believe that the social comparison phenomenon is more important now than ever. New media, including Twitter, Facebook, and Instagram, allow fans to feel close to celebrities. Naturally, I follow Gwyneth on Twitter. I hear from her every once in a while—she recently told me she was hanging with the fashion designer Jason Wu—but she isn't a frequent tweeter, especially compared to, say, the king of Twitter, Justin Bieber. As I write this, Bieber has about 47 million followers. (Think about that number. That is more than the population of California, Argentina, Australia, or Canada.) He has tweeted a remarkable twenty-four thousand times. That is about 3.3 million characters (assuming slightly fewer than 140 per tweet)—more than *War and Peace* has. Though not quite Tolstoyian in his literary sophistication, the Bieb can produce.

By the way, Katy Perry has almost fifty million followers, more than anyone, and Lady Gaga, forty-one million. Barack Obama, a man with stuff to tweet about, has a mere forty million.

This kind of new media presence creates an artificial closeness with celebrities. It makes us feel that celebrities are regular folks who live just around the cybercorner. One day, for example, Bieber told me by means of his Twitter feed that it was "a great Sunday so far" and that he was attending an "amazing sermon" that made him "break down." (I pictured him hunched in a pew and tweeting on his phone with tears in his eyes.) Even though the images of beauty projected by celebrity culture are as removed from reality as ever, or in fact more so, this virtual closeness makes it easier and more natural for us all to make comparisons. "Celebrities used to be glamorous and more removed. It was fantasy. Now, through social media, they feel closer, more real, and their world seems more attainable," Nancy Etcoff told me. Etcoff, a psychologist at Harvard Medical School, agrees that social media are having an impact on how individuals feel about their looks and how they present themselves. There is now pressure to always be "camera ready," Etcoff says. And celebrity culture produces the images that we all, consciously or unconsciously, seek to replicate. "Even the way people pose for the camera seems to have been influenced by celebrities and new media."

Ashley Mears agrees with Etcoff. She believes that new media have contributed to a growing gap between what is desired and what is attainable. "Perceptions of beauty are driven by a socially mediated desire for luxury and beauty. But it is just not obtainable," she says. "Especially since girls [models] are getting ever more slim, they are still so young, there is plastic surgery and airbrushing . . . all that is happening." Even the successful models Mears interviewed for her research "still feel inadequate," she says. And, increasingly, the images of these women are instantly available.

The research is still largely speculative, but some recent work supports the idea that social media are intensifying our compulsion to make social comparisons to unrealistic images. Studies show that the more personal the relationship is between an individual and a celebrity—in academic circles, this kind of illusory social-media-fueled intimacy is often called a parasocial relationship—the more likely it is to have an influence on things like body image and the likelihood of getting cosmetic surgery. For example, studies have shown that having a parasocial relationship with a celebrity who is "perceived as having a good body shape," as a relevant 2005 study by John Maltby and colleagues notes, "may lead to a poor body image."

There is ample evidence that noncelebrities appreciate the power of the images circulated through social media. A 2012 survey of facial plastic surgeons—the survey was undertaken by the American Academy of Facial Plastic and Reconstructive Surgery—found that 31 percent of the respondents saw an increase in requests for surgery as a result of social media photo sharing. Many people want to have plastic surgery in order to look good on the Internet. Indeed, the study reported that some patients specifically wanted plastic surgery "due to dissatisfaction with their image as displayed on social media sites." The survey concluded that patients are "more self aware of their looks because of social media," thus supporting both the idea that social media is intensifying the social comparison phenomenon and, as Etcoff suggests, that people want to be "camera ready." Not only are people comparing themselves to images of celebrities, they are altering their own image in order to compete in a perpetual Internet beauty competition, thereby heightening the importance of and—I am guessing here, as I could not find any data directly on point—narrowing the conception of beauty. It's as if we are all in an attractiveness arms race, an accelerating cycle of comparison and aesthetic modification that is moving us toward an attractiveness singularity that will cause the human race to be destroyed in a vast implosion of silicon, Botox, ab flexers, and eternal dissatisfaction. I exaggerate. Slightly.

Of course, new media such as Twitter also serve as forums for sharing ideas about social comparison. A 2013 study examined almost one thousand tweets sent before and during the *Victoria's Secret Fashion Show*. The authors found that many tweets demonstrated a harsh upward comparison to the fashion models. The lead author, psychologist Joan Chrisler, told me that she got the response she expected but was "struck by the tone of some of the tweets, particularly those that mentioned self-harm." She is not kidding. Here are some tweets Chrisler sent me to illustrate her point: "Eating a burrito then watching the Victoria's Secret Fashion

Show then crying while vomiting while slashing my wrists with a Gillette Venus"; "VICTORIA'S SECRET FASHION SHOW DRINKING GAME: drink every time you want to kill yourself"; and "The Victoria's Secret Fashion Show is pretty much the Super Bowl of bulimia isn't it?"

Chrisler agrees that "interacting" with celebrities through social media can create "a kind of faux intimacy," as she calls it. While she says more robust research is needed, she worries that the trend is harmful. "When we compare ourselves to our real friends, whom we know are not perfect, it might not be as stark or as painful a comparison as when we compare ourselves to our Facebook and Twitter 'friends' who look perfect in their carefully chosen photographs." And this, it seems, is exactly what happens. A study published after my exchange with Chrisler found a strong correlation for photo sharing on Facebook, body dissatisfaction, and a drive for thinness among adolescent girls. Facebook increases the opportunity to "self-objectify and make physical appearance comparisons" with other girls and celebrities. It should not be forgotten that easy access to a vast quantity of images of idealized humans is a relatively recent technological development. Constantly being exposed to high-definition pictures of beautiful celebrities is, in the modern world, taken for granted. They are simply a part of our everyday experience. But just a couple of hundred years ago, the only images available of other men or women were either the people themselves, physically present, or a painting or drawing of them. For most of the population, I bet, even high-quality versions of the latter were relatively rare. So your comparators were real humans. Sure, strolling the streets of, say, Stockholm can be pretty demoralizing to the average Canadian. (I am pretty sure Sweden has some kind of cruel beauty bylaw that banishes average-looking people to a colony north of the Arctic Circle.) But now our social comparators are rarely real. They are illusions created by pop culture.

ONE WONDERS WHAT the future will hold. As computer-generated imagery (CGI) technology increases in sophistication, will our comparators become completely removed from reality? Will they evolve from the largely fabricated (i.e., cosmetically enhanced, air-brushed, and genetically lucky celebrities) to the completely fabricated (i.e., a computer-generated image)? There are hints this could happen. In the fall of 2013, an incredibly lifelike computer-generated image of a ten-year-old girl named Sweetie was used by a Dutch children's charity to lure and capture more than one thousand pedophiles. The men thought the image was of a real girl, so real that they offered to pay her to perform sex acts. (Some men reportedly asked her if she had a younger sister.) The sting operation, which did not involve law enforcement officials, was conducted by the children's advocacy charity Terre des Hommes. The case is disturbing, but it serves to highlight the power of CGI. More than twenty thousand men tried to contact this nonexistent girl.

TO BE CLEAR, I am *not* bashing the idea of losing weight or adopting a healthy, active lifestyle. On the contrary, losing a significant amount of weight and keeping it off is a tremendous achievement. We live in a society where approximately 60 percent of the population is overweight and about one-third obese. This is a serious public health issue, perhaps the defining health challenge of our generation. But the message that flows from the celebrity universe rarely has anything to do with health. The message is almost always about appearance. It is about looking great.

Emme looks great. It is no surprise that she has *twice* been named one of *People's* 50 Most Beautiful People and was *Glamour's* woman of the year in 1997. She has that aura of a beautiful person: that effortless center-of-attention pull. Indeed, moments after I meet Emme—she is one of those famous individuals who have dispensed with a last name—I find myself reflecting on the beauty research I have been discussing. *Do Emme's great energy and confidence make her more beautiful, or did beauty give her more confidence, which in turn made her more beautiful?*

I am hanging out with Emme in her New York office, where she is coordinating her latest project, Emme Nation. She is the world's most famous, and arguably successful, plus-size model. She is tall and looks like she could still be an elite rower, which was what she was doing when, as she tells it, she "fell into modeling." While she is still involved in the fashion world, her career focus has changed. One of Emme's current goals is to advocate for a healthy body image, a cause she is uniquely qualified to champion.

"Celebrity culture and the beauty industry are designed to make you feel bad," Emme says. And, sadly, these social forces seem to be winning. A 2011 survey of American women found a staggering 97 percent had at least one "I hate my body" thought each day, and on average women have thirteen negative thoughts about their body daily. (This frequency, incidentally, is just slightly less than the number of times men think about sex in a day, which is not, contrary to the urban myth, once every seven seconds.)

Because self-improvement is not about health or well-being, we are all caught, men included, in a bizarre health-beauty paradox. Our primary motivation for self-improvement—as sold to us by popular culture and, I think, as wired in our brains—is to achieve aesthetic changes to our body. But a combination of biological predisposition, circumstance, and the ravages inflicted by time means that the vast majority of us are incapable of achieving the aesthetic ideal. As a result, we end up discouraged and unhappy. Most worryingly, perhaps, we are dissuaded from undertaking the kind of activities that may, in the long term, have significant health and happiness benefits.

There is a good deal of research on this dilemma. One study, published in 2013, examined more than five thousand pages of popular women's health and fitness magazines, including *Fitness, Self, Shape, Health,* and *Prevention.* The researchers found, no surprise, weight loss and body shaping to be major topics, taking up more than one-fifth of all content. More important, however, the focus of the articles was largely on appearance as opposed to health—that is, they pushed the idea that the reason to diet and exercise is to look good, not to be healthy.

The articles I read in *People* almost always focused on looks. "Miranda's Brand-New Look!," "Hottest Diets!," and more. Moreover, they were often associated with unscientific advice about how to lose weight (cleansing! juicing!). Incidentally, the number of articles about losing weight after giving birth astounded me. Readers must love this stuff.

That looks are a central theme probably surprises no one: we are evolutionarily wired to focus on and care about appearances. Indeed, research has consistently supported the idea that this is one of the primary motivations for people to diet and exercise. Even older individuals—people at a stage in life when, you would think, they would be pretty focused on health—recognize that appearance is a stronger motivator. A study from 2002 involved in-depth interviews of women aged sixty-one to ninety-two. These were not spring chickens. Even for this group, vanity ruled. "Many of the women suggest that while the health benefits of weight loss are often the stated reason for losing weight," the author notes, "the perceived appearance dividends are the key motivation behind altering one's body weight in later life."

So what? If people are exercising and dieting and focusing on themselves, who cares if appearance is the primary motivation? Who cares if they are doing it because they want to look like Gwyneth, Jennifer, Selena, Brad, or Channing, so long as they are doing it? This is a complicated issue. On the one hand, there is a body of research that tells us how counterproductive the focus on appearance can be. A study of more than two hundred women, published in 2012, found that appearance-based motives for weight loss and exercise are associated with a range of negative outcomes, including body image concerns. Other studies have shown that dieting for appearance, as opposed to health, is associated with binge eating and frequent (and unsuccessful) dieting. Those who are dieting to improve their looks are also less likely to be happy with their appearance than those dieting for health (admittedly, the direction of causation is unclear). They are also more likely to be stressed out by the dieting process. That is, dieting is especially psychologically taxing when the goal is appearance and not health. And still other studies have found that people focusing on looks are less likely to stay motivated and, as a result, are less likely to adopt a long-term, sustainable healthy lifestyle.

On the other hand, some research shows that vanity can motivate healthy changes in behavior. The implication is that public health advocates should simply embrace our obsession with appearance. We have seen this tactic work with antismoking campaigns. When people are scared by pictures that show the aesthetic damage wrought by tobacco, some try to quit. Other studies have found that if you want people to avoid sun exposure, messages about appearance (unsightly wrinkles) are more powerful than messages about health (dying of cancer). The effectiveness of this approach has led some health-care professionals to advocate its use in other contexts, such as in the promotion of fruit and vegetable consumption (currently, fewer than a third of us eat enough). And a few studies have found that, at least for a relatively short period and in specific circumstances, being motivated by appearance can help people achieve weight-loss goals.

While I can see the logic of leveraging looks to achieve health goals, I am skeptical about both the long-term effectiveness and social sustainability of the approach. Too many studies have found that people who are motivated by appearance are less likely to stick with a health-related behavior. Vanity might be a good hook, but research tells us that over time, emphasizing health and the intrinsic worth of a healthy lifestyle is the better approach.

I also have another problem with the do-it-for-looks strategy. This approach would seem to subtly legitimize both the *People* ethos that self-improvement is about looks and the feel-bad-about-your-looks message emanating from celebrity culture generally. The approach invites social comparison. (To cite one example, a *People* cover lauds Kate Middleton's postbaby bod. So, if you've just had a baby and don't look like Kate, get to work!) It suggests that appearance and body modification— and, ya know, looking like a celeb—*should* be viewed as the central goal. The do-it-for-looks strategy of achieving better health would, I speculate, increase the rotational velocity and soul-sucking power of the celebrity-established-beauty-standard vortex.

Here is a list of just a few of the evidence-based benefits of exercise that have absolutely *nothing* to do with appearance: better sleep, better sex, better memory, better mental health, protection against dementia, protection against the adverse effects of stress, an association with a reduced suicide risk, higher grades for kids, and, of course, all the well-known benefits associated with cardiovascular health and the reduction of risk for various cancers. A similar nothing-to-do-with-looks list could be produced for the benefits of a nutritious and calorie-appropriate diet. But all these benefits, no matter how well advertised by public health educators, seem unlikely to compete successfully as a source of motivation with even one Instagram picture of Gwyneth in a Stella McCartney bikini, an image generating significant pop-culture buzz as I write. In the photo, Gwyneth is leaping through the air wearing a faux leopard-skin two-piece and a big gee-don't-I-look-great smile. (And, to be fair, she certainly does.) Naturally, commentary on the image consistently affirms the lifestyle-for-looks mythology. "This is what 5-day workouts during the week and a strict diet will get you!" declares Perezhilton.com. "Looks like all those juice cleanses and a strict no-carb diet has [*sic*] paid off for Gwyneth Paltrow," says the *Huffington Post*. If health-care providers, health systems, schools, parents, and public health officials don't continue to wave the health-message flag, who will? Perez? Another problem is that if we are told looks are the goal, taking shortcuts, even unhealthy shortcuts, might seem perfectly sensible.

Currently, approximately 6 percent of high school boys take steroids in order to build muscle mass, according to a 2012 study published in the journal *Pediatrics*. That number is astonishing on its own, but even more shocking is that nonathletes are just as likely as athletes to use these dangerous and illegal substances. Clearly, kids often are taking steroids simply to achieve a particular look. This study found that steroid use in the study group is not driven by school sports but by factors such as "media messages and social norms of behavior more broadly." Another study, published in *Pediatrics* in 2014, found that more than 20 percent of gay teenage boys had used steroids. Again, the authors speculated that this is driven almost entirely by the desire to achieve an idealized male physique.

Of course, another shortcut to body modification without the justification of health benefits is cosmetic surgery, an increasingly popular practice that, as I have discussed, has been linked directly to celebrity culture. There also has been a recent, rapid growth in bariatric surgery tourism—that is, people traveling to countries to get weight-loss surgery. These are often individuals who do not want to wait for, or do not meet the clinical criteria to get, the surgery in their home country. Many clinics in other countries explicitly offer these services to teenagers. The fact is that media portrayals of weight-loss surgery promote a false sense of what the surgery can achieve (a 2013 study by colleagues at the University of Alberta, for example, found these reports to be both inaccurate and overly simplistic), often with reference to celebrity success stories like those of Randy Jackson, Sharon Osbourne, Al Roker, Roseanne Barr, and Star Jones. In reality, these are potentially dangerous procedures that not infrequently lead to serious postoperative complications. And though bariatric surgery can, from a health perspective, be highly effective, it does not always lead to the expected aesthetic result.

"Television shows, popular magazines, and other popular media have probably contributed to the normalization and routinization of bariatric surgery. Celebrities who undergo bariatric surgery generate intense media coverage," Leigh Turner tells me. Turner, a professor at the Center for Bioethics and the School of Public Health at the University of Minnesota, has studied the ethical issues associated with the bariatric surgery industry and is concerned about how these services are marketed. "Patients can gain access to surgical procedures that will likely be of no benefit to them and can put them at significant risk of harm," Turner says. In other words, these international services—which often do not include the long-term clinical and lifestyle support necessary to make bariatric surgery a success—are often a dangerous shortcut to nowhere.

Cutting Through the Confusion

Celebrity culture spews out such a vast amount of pseudoscientific noise that a bit of science-informed clarity is desperately needed. Numerous studies have confirmed that despite the obvious wrongheadedness of so much of the extant beauty and health advice, people remain thoroughly confused about what actually works. Moreover, in an era when obesity has emerged as one of the biggest public health concerns, and when issues associated with body image—including some eating disorders—appear to be on the rise, celebrity culture emphasizes precisely the wrong solutions. Instead of embracing a healthy, sustainable lifestyle that focuses on long-term well-being, celebrity culture focuses on and promotes short-term aesthetic goals that are, for 99 percent of the population, impossible to achieve. Allow me to provide a few broad conclusions that tie together some of the central evidence-based themes of what I have been saying about celebrity culture in this section. They are obvious and simple, but that is, in part, the whole point.

Weight-loss and diet gimmicks never work and are rarely supported by actual science. This may seem an overstatement, but both history (can you name just *one* diet fad that has panned out, long term?) and the best available research support it. And don't be fooled by the celebrity status of the endorsers, the medical credentials of the inventors, or the pseudoscientific jargon that so often accompanies the claims. The best diet is the simple, balanced diet we have known about for decades.

All novel and apparently simple solutions to vague health problems are likely bogus. Alas, the human body is complex. It is rare that we can "fix" an ailment or condition through the use of one novel, "breakthrough" intervention. Be suspicious of all simple (and scientifically unsubstantiated) diagnostic tests and quick-fix solutions (vitamins, supplements, special diets), particularly when they are aimed at relatively amorphous and subjectively assessed problems (anxiety, fatigue, stress).

You don't need to detox, cleanse, juice, hyperhydrate, supplement, etc. This one is easy. There is simply no good evidence for any of these health trends, and for some—like extreme detoxes, high doses of vitamins, and colon cleanses—the evidence tells us they can be harmful. In fact, if some new health trend emerges, no matter how enticing and logical it may seem, I can almost guarantee it will lack solid science. These alternative approaches to nutrition never work. So start with that assumption and you will likely be correct 99.9 percent of the time.

There is little reliable science to support many of the claims that flow from the beauty and antiaging industry. Given the size of this industry, I was astounded by the lack of good, independent research. The beauty industry efficacy bias—BIEB—really does dominate this world. You can disregard almost everything that flows from this industry. Save your money. Few products and procedures will have a dramatic impact. Even in the context of cosmetic surgery—which can, obviously, result in significant physical changes—the impact, both aesthetically and psychologically, is likely to be more modest than expected.

Celebrity culture encourages a range of unhealthy behavior. Sunbathing, extreme diets, ingestion of unnecessary vitamins, and potentially ill-advised cosmetic surgery are just a few of the examples that fall into this category. I don't think celebrities do this on purpose. As the experiences of people like Kyla Wise demonstrate, celebrities are subject to the same twisting forces about beauty and health that afflict the rest of us. Arguably, they are more vulnerable. This is a systemic phenomenon, not some celebrity-driven conspiracy. But the evidence tells us that, whether we know it or not, celebrity culture has an impact.

Celebrity culture helps to set unrealistic beauty norms and makes us feel bad about ourselves and our looks. While the data on the long-term impact of celebrity culture in some domains may still be iffy, most evidence supports the spirit of this proposition, particularly for the short term and for individuals who are already at risk. Indeed, we are likely biologically wired and socially encouraged to constantly compare ourselves to other humans. This, in our media-saturated world, often means the ridiculously attractive images of celebrities. And new media tools, such as Facebook, Twitter, and Instagram, increase both the power and frequency of such comparisons. But we are comparing ourselves to illusions. This does little to contribute to our day-to-day happiness.

Celebrity culture encourages uncritical, magical thinking. One of the most destructive and worrisome aspects of celebrity culture's grip on society is that it seems to facilitate a pseudoscientific approach to health and beauty. An endless parade of celebrities either peddles scientifically unsupportable ideas or—through actions, images, and statements—endorses pseudoscientific products and approaches to health and beauty. All this noise is often accompanied by an authoritative rhetoric—for example, Gwyneth's cleanse. But rarely is any real science involved. Testimonials and anecdote are *not* evidence. In fact, one essential function of the scientific method is to cut through the bias created by personal perceptions and the persuasive force of anecdote. When reviewing the claims associated with new health and beauty products, we must look for good, supporting data.

The Science-Informed Six

Celebrity culture is such a powerful and pervasive force that it likely has an impact on our perceptions and beliefs even when we don't recognize it. I have had numerous gluten-free, juicing, cleansed, detoxified friends and acquaintances tell me, without a hint of irony, some version of this: "Only an idiot would listen to celebrities." But the influence is subtle and hard to ignore. Celebrity culture leverages our biologically predetermined love affair with beauty, helping to perpetuate an aesthetic angst that can never be resolved, especially by the useless products and advice that flow from the celebrity maw. We should constantly remind ourselves of the existence of these cultural forces and biological predispositions. Perhaps say a little mantra: *We should not let celebrity lies defy the science-informed six.* (Sure, I'm not Jay Z or Eminem . . . or, even, Vanilla Ice, but it works.) From a health perspective, these six steps are well known and time tested:

1. Don't smoke, and drink alcohol in moderation.
2. Stay active, stand often, exercise regularly, and include some vigorous activities.
3. Eat a balanced and calorie-appropriate diet that includes lots of fruits and vegetables, whole grains, lean protein (such as fish, chicken, beans, and nuts), and healthy fats (such as olive oil); avoid bad fats (those of the trans variety).
4. Maintain a healthy weight (tough, I know).
5. Wear sunscreen.
6. Get an appropriate amount of sleep (which, for most, is between seven and nine hours).

That is it. Everything else is either total baloney or of such marginal value when compared to the impact of these actions as to be nearly irrelevant. For example, if you smoke or don't exercise, worrying about eating organic food is like Wile E. Coyote using that tiny, broken umbrella to minimize the effects of a house-size boulder falling on his head.

Celebrity culture, at best, is selling us a tiny, broken umbrella.

Part II

The Illusion That You Too Can Be a Celebrity

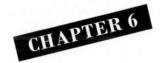

Dreams of Fame
and Fortune

"This is such a great album!" I declare to no one in particular.

This is my reflexive, near-Pavlovian, know-it-all response to hearing the opening bars of "Wouldn't It Be Nice," the first song on the Beach Boys'—or, if we are being honest, Brian Wilson's—remarkable *Pet Sounds*.

I am standing at the counter in a Paris bookshop with my teenage son, Adam. The album is playing over the store's sound system. Adam has been subjected to a lifetime of my music-related pontifications, so all I get in response is an raised eyebrow and a half-smile that tells me, "Yep, Dad, I know, you like this album. And by the way, you are kind of embarrassing."

But someone else is listening. "This *is* a great album," the cashier says in accent-free English. He is young and hip. The kind of guy you would not be surprised to find working in, well, a cool Parisian bookstore.

"It is amazing how many current bands have adopted this sound," I say in an effort to stimulate further discussion. "Like, for example, the band Beach House. Much of their stuff has a big *Pet Sounds* vibe."

"Funny you should say that," the hip book salesman replies. "I was the drummer for Beach House."

To truly appreciate the otherworldly weirdness of this coincidence, consider the following: Both Adam and I love Beach House. All the group's albums have ended up on "best of" lists. From the outside looking in, Beach House seems like a commercially successful outfit. The band has played on *David Letterman* and regularly sells out medium-size venues all over the world. When I think of a "Beach House lifestyle," I think tour buses, personal assistants, and nice hotels. A rock 'n' roll existence. So you won't be surprised to know that my first thought is, *Yeah, right, I'm sure you were the drummer for Beach House.* And that my second thought, which comes after some further banter that had the not-so-well-hidden goal of confirming the veracity of the drummer's claim, is, *What the hell is a bona fide rock star doing working in a bookstore?*

Dreams of Fame and Fortune

Twenty-five years ago the top five career ambitions of grade-school children were teacher, banker, doctor, scientist, and vet. Now, according to a recent UK survey, they are, in descending order of awesomeness: sports star, pop star, actor, astronaut, and lawyer. While the choice of lawyer may seem reasonably sensible (hey, I'm a lawyer!), I suspect most of these kids have no interest in being a real lawyer. They aren't dreaming of working ninety hours a week on personal-injury cases for a soul-sucking law firm. They don't want to drag their butts out of bed at 5:30 a.m. to get in a few extra billable hours. They don't want to babysit two hundred or so mind-numbing client files. They want to be the slick, fast-talking, well-dressed, sexy TV-drama version of a lawyer. (I can personally confirm that this version does not exist.)

The dream of celebrity and fame endures well into late adolescence. Another UK study, involving more than one thousand sixteen-year-olds, found that more than half had fame as their primary career goal. Other UK research has found that, in 2006, 16 percent of sixteen- to nineteen-year-olds believed they were going to be famous. Eleven percent were ready to quit school to pursue this goal. My daughter Alison was sufficiently surprised by these numbers that she queried her twenty-six ninth-grade classmates about their aspirations. More than 50 percent told her that they were hoping for a celebrity-oriented profession. Six saw themselves becoming actors; five, professional athletes; and several, film directors. Only one in this class of relatively affluent children wanted to be a scientist, which is a bit ironic, given that the school sits blocks from my university's huge new biomedical research building. One student is hoping to be a doctor, and another is aiming for teaching—drama, naturally. One said he wanted to be an explosives expert. (Is that a job?)

Jake Halpern surveyed 650 US teenagers for his book, *Fame Junkies*. A remarkable 43.4 percent aspired to be an assistant to a "very famous singer or movie star." In comparison, 23.7 percent said they wanted to be "the president of a great university like Harvard or Yale," 13.6 percent saw themselves as "a United States Senator," 9.8 percent as a "Navy Seal," and 9.5 percent as chief of a major company. Think about that. Four out of ten teenagers would rather get coffee, make appointments, and pick up dry cleaning for a celebrity than have their own prestigious and rewarding career!

The bottom line: fame and celebrity status are now *the* dominant ambitions. Kids just want to be famous. And a growing body of research supports this finding. A 2011 study, for example, found that fame was the number-one cultural value of children aged ten to twelve. The kids in this study were asked to think about their future and the traits they would like to possess: being famous was their top choice. Indeed, the abstract notion of fame—the desire simply to be known by a large number of strangers—as a future goal ranked well above being kind, successful, having love and acceptance, or even being rich. And perhaps most interesting, the researcher found that none of the children in the study, not a single one, mentioned a particular skill or talent associated with the concept of fame. Not one said he or she wanted to excel at a sport or at acting. Another study asked ten-year-olds what they believed would be "the very best thing in the world." The number-one answer: "Being a celebrity." "Friends" ranked seventh.

One of the most comprehensive research projects on point was conducted in Tasmania, Australia, in 2011. The researchers asked more than
one thousand primary-school children about their hopes and dreams.
Once again, fame and celebrity were the overriding themes. A few young-
sters were aiming for prime minister, but, in general, the kids wanted to
be entertainment and sports stars. For part of the study they were asked
to draw a picture of a leaf with their hopes for the future written on it.
Some were general. Versions of the nebulous "I want to be famous" were
common. Others were pretty specific. One sixth-grade boy, for example,
said he wanted "to be an actor and to live in Los Angeles and to have a
lovely wife and two children living the high life." (That does sound like a
mighty fine lifestyle.) Many kids saw music as their portal to fame. Here
are two of my favorite quotes, both from sixth-grade boys: "My hope is
that my band makes it into the big bucks and famous. Rock on!" and "I
would like to be rich with a big mansion. To become a well-known musician that plays in a band."

IN THIS PART OF THE BOOK, I'll try to shed some light on the reality of the
fame game and the drive for celebrity. Everything is an illusion. Not only
is there no pot of gold at the end of the rainbow (well, there is, rarely,
a pot, but it usually isn't filled with the promised, happiness-inducing
gold), but the rainbow isn't real. It is a projection created by the market,
the media, our own cognitive and biologically determined predisposition, and our hopes and dreams. Moreover, believing in the existence of
the celebrity rainbow has numerous adverse consequences.

It may seem, at least initially, that this section is a real downer. Pulling the curtain back on the illusion of celebrity can come off a bit frosty.
My younger brother, Sean, once was sent home from kindergarten for
running a recess seminar on his "there is no Santa Claus" theory, which
was largely based on the hypothesis that Christmas is a capitalist plot
designed to sell lots of toys. (I wonder who forced these radical ideas into
his impressionable five-year-old brain.) I don't want to be *that* guy now.

I don't want to kill Santa Claus. Big dreams, even if unrealistic, are fun and can play an important social role. Plus, I can completely relate to the fantasy of fame. I devoted a significant part of my young adult life to the pursuit of rock 'n' roll stardom.

But, more important, I believe the message of this section is liberating. Ideally, it will release us from the grip of celebrity-fueled ambitions and the social expectations that come with them. I hope it allows us to make more informed choices as individuals, parents, or community members. More broadly, I hope it highlights the pernicious effect of celebrity culture on our values and our conception of the good life.

One can become a celebrity a whole bunch of ways. There are famous authors (though not many, and the benefits conferred on them by fame usually are modest). There are famous politicians (though that doesn't seem like a fun kind of fame). And there are even famous scientists (again, not many). In this era, however, I think most people associate fame and celebrity with several fairly specific activities: music, acting, sports, and, um, nothing (the relatively new famous-for-being-famous gig). These are the avenues to fame most often mentioned by children and adolescents. Rock star! Movie star! Sports star! So these will be the areas I will focus on in my attempt to show how illusory they really are.

Of course, young people are not the only ones yearning for celebrity status. Other research tells us that fame remains the number-one goal for a significant number of adults, hence the steady stream of reality show applicants. A recent US survey found that fame and celebrity increasingly have become what people view as the American dream. It is never too late to be famous, I guess. As I mentioned, I held on to my rock star dreams well into my twenties. In fact, I think my twenty-sixth birthday was my most depressing, far more so than when I turned thirty or forty. Those later birthdays breezed by without a drop of age-related despondency. But my twenty-sixth was the year that I had a full-on existential crisis. It was the year I realized I would never be the front man of a monstrously successful and critically acclaimed rock band. That dream, alas, was dead.

It's not just kids whose imaginations are fired up by the prospect of fame. Many parents see some form of celebrity—athlete, actor, or pop star—as the most desirable career option for their children. For some, seeking celebrity has become a central family activity, one that consumes a significant amount of their financial resources and their time. Is all this striving, whether for yourself or your children, folly? Can we really all become celebrities if we just keep dreaming big and reaching for the stars?

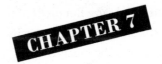

So You Want to Be a Star?

Rock Star!

My flight to the South by Southwest (SXSW) music festival in Austin, Texas, was nonstop from New York. Judging by the number of guitar cases, the quantity of DJ gear, the predominance of I-wish-I-didn't-have-to-get-up expressions on people's faces, and the answers to a few random queries, the boarding area at JFK was overflowing with musicians. There was a smattering of fans, business executives, music lawyers, and people involved in music promotion, but mostly it was bedraggled individuals wearing attire that unimaginatively advertised their musical affiliation: hip-hop, alt country, rock 'n' roll, retro punk, ironic quirky pop. The plane at the gate next to our flight was heading to Florida. The slow-moving passenger line was peppered with wheelchairs, Bermuda shorts, and polo shirts. The contrast with the hipster caravan I was about to join could not have been starker. One line filled with retirees, the other with people who probably rarely think about that kind of late-life lifestyle.

SXSW is billed as the world's largest music conference or, as its website declares, the "biggest and most anticipated convergence of all things music." More than two thousand "official" musical acts are playing at hundreds of venues—large, medium, and rumpus-room-ish in dimension—throughout the downtown core. The roster includes well-established big-name bands, up-and-coming acts, and bands that are new but have lots of buzz. (I heard the word *buzz* hundreds of times while at SXSW, as in: "no buzz," "buzzless," "about to catch some buzz," "no point in coming unless you have buzz," and the much-coveted "buzz band.") There are also hundreds, perhaps thousands, of unofficial acts that play in unofficial (rough, closet-size) venues.

While the music is the focus and the public draw, the music industry people I spoke with told me that SXSW is really a big schmoozefest industry party. Given this fine mandate, it seemed an ideal place to explore the state of the music industry and its role in the celebrity game. Specifically, I wanted to explore the current status of the celebrity musician. Is the rock star job still available? And, more broadly, can you get rich and famous in music?

My guide for the event is a good friend, C.J. Murdoch—aka Cecil Frena, Edmonton's electropop music wiz and leader of the one-man band Born Gold. C.J.'s career path might be considered eccentric by some. He was a rising star in the world of legal academia. He obtained a law degree from the University of Alberta, was a researcher for the university's Health Law Institute, published a number of well-received academic articles, was given a fellowship at Stanford University, and, just a few years ago, gave it all up. C.J. went all in. He doesn't do music as a hobby or as a part-time job. He is a full-time struggling musician. And wow! The vast majority of professional musicians do *struggle*.

In March 2013 the Canandian Independent Music Association released a comprehensive report on the economic impact of the music industry. The message was pretty clear. If getting rich and famous is your goal, pick a different profession. The average income for an independent musician in Canada is $7,228 per year. Yes, per *year*. That is less than half the amount the Canadian government has set as the poverty line for single people and thousands less than the average income threshold for poverty for single people in the United States. And we aren't talking about garage bands whose members are attending the local community college and living at home with Mom and Dad. The average age of these impoverished Canadian minstrels was thirty-nine (I suppose they could still be at home with Mom and Dad), and the average size audience they played to was well over seven hundred. These are people putting in full-time or near full-time hours. These are real, touring, hardworking, professional musicians. The kind you pay good money to see. The kind who play at SXSW, have cool T-shirts (an important source of income), and that you hear on commercial radio.

As I went from venue to venue—using C.J. as my backstage pass—I ran these numbers by various musicians, both experienced and inexperienced, from all over North America and got the same that's-about-right reaction. Some were initially shocked, many laughed at the absurdity of their situation, but after a bit of reflection, everyone agreed that the depressing numbers provided by the Canadian Independent Music Association rang true. You might be thinking, sure, independent musicians don't make much. They are, after all, *independent* musicians. In order to catch the celebrity-propelling brass ring, you need to sign a record deal with a big label. Well, you're both right and wrong.

It's true that the chance of making it really big without industry money is remote. One analysis of the UK music scene concluded that your chance of financial "success" (modestly defined as making the national average income for *one year*) without a major record deal is next to zero. After considering the number of "serious" musicians in the United Kingdom, and the money generated from paying gigs and downloads, the author concluded that the chance of making an average income for just one year was a stupefyingly unlikely 0.0025 percent. But even if you snag an industry record deal, there is absolutely no guarantee you will make any money or get close to achieving celebrity.

Moses Avalon, a well-known music industry expert and commentator, has written several books on the music scene, including the often-referenced *Confessions of a Record Producer*. He is a fearless skeptic and crusader for artists' rights, so he seemed to be an ideal person to approach about the reality of rock 'n' roll stardom. More important, not long ago he did an impressive analysis of the very issue I was exploring: the chances of making it big with a major label deal.

Avalon estimates that of the 43,000 submissions that go to major labels each year, only one in 2,149 will make it through a multiple-album deal, which is probably what is required to achieve what he calls a "quitting your day job" standard of living. Put another way: only .047 percent will have anything close to a stable career. (Many commentators think that Avalon's already-bleak number is in fact *too* optimistic, because they figure the number of submissions, if you include all the basement-tape demos, is much larger.) While these odds are terrifyingly slim, Avalon notes that they are better than trying to stay indie. According to his analysis, based on the "raw odds," as he says, of selling about five thousand units for several albums in a row, what are the chances of "quitting your day job" indie success? 1:477,000! As Avalon notes, it may not be one in a million, but from the perspective of a struggling indie artist, it might as well be. When I called to ask about his analysis, he immediately displayed his pull-no-punches approach to life. He said he didn't like my first question about the chances of making it celebrity big. "I don't want to tell you how to do an interview . . . but what the hell do you mean [by] 'celebrity rock star'? Every singer in a band thinks he is a rock star."

Good point.

"Look, it has *always* been near impossible to become a true, Jagger-style rock star," Avalon continued. "That is a billion-to-one phenomenon. It just doesn't happen."

OF COURSE, THERE ARE many paths to fame and fortune in the music industry. Thanks to shows such as *American Idol*, the way can seem tremendously short and spectacularly direct. The premise of the show, and all its imitators, is that contestants have the chance to realize their dreams instantly. But what is the likelihood that a show such as *Idol* will propel a person to celebrity status? Pretty darn small.

My oldest son, Adam, analyzed the careers of the *Idol* contestants who finished in the top twelve in the first five seasons. I asked Adam to do this for two reasons. First, he's cheap labor. Second, I wanted to access his teenage sensibilities in the assessment of whether a contestant was successful. I wanted to know if, through the eyes of a media-saturated teenager, a given *Idol* contestant was celebrity big. For each contestant, Adam looked through Twitter, iTunes, and other relevant websites (e.g., Internet Movie Database). He looked for stories about their careers, record contracts, involvement in Broadway productions, and the like. We then worked together to give each top-finishing *Idol* contestant a ranking, from a Carrie Underwood high (as the most successful *Idol* contestant ever, she gets a rank of 10) to singing-on-a-cruise-ship low. What did we find? Though many *Idol* finalists are working in the entertainment industry, few have found anything close to what could be considered big-time success. Of the fifty-eight finalists (the first season had ten) we tracked, Kelly Clarkson, Clay Aiken, Ruben Studdard, Jennifer Hudson, Fantasia Barrino, Carrie Underwood, Chris Daughtry, Katherine McPhee, and Taylor Hicks rated as an 8 or above. These are the few who have relatively broad name recognition and reasonably solid careers. Others, such as Mandisa from season five (Christian music) and Constantine Maroulis from season four (musical theater) are doing well, but I think this is a fair list of the contestants who can be classified as truly successful by industry standards. (One could argue that we were overly generous in our assessment of Hicks, Studdard, and Barrino—none of my kids had ever heard of them. Ditto my kids' friends.)

It is difficult to find the exact number of people who try out for *Idol*, but estimates range from 50,000 to 100,000 per season. So, altogether, approximately 200,000 to 300,000 people likely auditioned in those first five years. This means there is about a 9 in 250,000 chance of celebrity success through *Idol*. Once again, this means, from the perspective of a practical assessment of your odds, that your chance might as well be zero. Even if we take an extremely conservative approach and guesstimate that only 1 out of every 100 who audition sing well enough to be in the mix, and suppose for the sake of argument that you are one of them, this still translates into about a 0.36 percent chance of a career that will fall somewhere between Taylor Hicks and Carrie Underwood. Even the top 1 percent of *Idol* contestants have a slim chance of celebrity success.

Of course, we need to be careful in our definition of "success"—a point I will return to. Here, I am talking about making it celebrity big, not some form of artistic success—which is, of course, a critical distinction, particularly in the world of reality TV.

I interviewed Lisa Leuschner, an *Idol* semifinalist from season three. The woman can sing. Indeed, she has been called "the most prematurely, unjustly eliminated contestant in show history"; her performance of "Sweet Thing" was an *Idol* standout. But despite her obvious talent and comfort on the stage, the judges voted her off the show. (It is worth noting that on an earlier show one of the judges—Simon Cowell, no surprise—commented on her weight, suggesting she was too big to be an *Idol* winner. It is unclear whether this is the reason she was voted off.) Despite this, she isn't bitter about her *Idol* ride, mostly because she seems to have a remarkably clear-headed appreciation—at least for someone who has invested time in *American Idol*—of the nature of the music industry. This is the result, no doubt, of her extensive pre-*Idol* experience as a working singer. I asked her why so many people continue to audition for the show.

"Many of the kids on *Idol* [are] caught up in the star thing," Leuschner tells me. "Many have no idea what it is like to be a musician. It is not an easy job. It is hard work. But I have no regrets. I feel blessed to be a working singer. That's who I am."

Leuschner continues to be employed—performing mostly blues and gospel. As of this writing (and I am streaming her amazing voice as I type these words), she is touring with the band Foreverland, a tribute to Michael Jackson. Leuschner's experience highlights a point that should be abundantly clear by now: raw ability and hard work are absolutely no guarantee of success on *Idol* or in the music industry generally. If you define success as doing something you love, Leuschner is doing just fine. The problem is that in the world of celebrity wannabes, success is rarely defined in such sensible terms. Anything other than stardom can be cast as a failure.

I ask another former *Idol* contestant, Martin Kerr, about our culture's fame-focused standard of success. Kerr finished in the top sixteen of the now-defunct Canadian version of the show and has since carved out a solid singing career. While far from famous, Kerr tells me he has attained what most would consider a middle-class lifestyle. And he has achieved this not by selling CDs or touring the world but by playing "local farmers' markets, churches, schools, house concerts, weddings, festivals, charity and corporate events, stuff that many musicians don't even consider doing." He is entirely satisfied with his musical career and is frustrated because most people view success in terms of fame and fortune. "I think it's strange that we judge success in music by a different yardstick than other industries," Kerr notes. "If you work in IT and make a good living at it, people consider you a success. They don't say, 'Keep trying' or 'I hope you make it someday' because you're not Bill Gates. But if you do the same in music, people say exactly those things until they've seen you on MTV."

Movie Star!

The best estimates I could find suggest that there are about thirty thousand professional actors in New York City. At the same time, according to some calculations, there are about eight hundred good jobs available to them, ranging from Off-Broadway bit parts to steady chorus line work to leads in major productions. Not a lot of jobs for an awful lot of actors. And the thirty thousand figure includes only those actors who are a member of one of the relevant unions—individuals who are generally experienced and arguably employable. If you include all the other actors struggling to get a paying gig who are not yet part of a union—assuming the 3:1 ratio suggested to me by several actors—then we are closing in on a final count of about a hundred thousand desperate thespians. I met one of them in a bar overlooking Union Square.

Ramesh Ganeshram is a good-looking guy. He clearly satisfies the actor-must-be-at-least-kinda-hot criterion. Also, he has a hard-to-pin-down ethnicity. Is he Indian? Arab? Ethiopian? (As he later joked, "I can play everything from evil terrorist to nonthreatening friendly ethnic neighbor to everything in between—it is a good time for a guy like me!"). These luck-of-the-draw genetic characteristics must, I suppose (somewhat uncomfortably), help to set him apart from at least a few of the one hundred thousand.

Ganeshram gives me a warm hello and firm handshake. He seems to be an ideal case study for this book. He is your typical working actor, still struggling to "make it big."

We settle into our booth, and he starts telling me about his career, the various acting schools and classes he has attended, the theater work he has done, the bit parts he has played in independent movies, and so on, but he seems more than a little distracted. It turns out that he had an audition earlier that day for the popular NBC-TV show *Law and Order: SVU*. It was a small part but a good one. It was network TV, paid real money, and would be a great addition to his resume. He wanted it. Badly. It was going to be tough for him to relax, he informs me after a long soul-centering sigh, until he hears how the audition went. This is understandable. I order a beer. He orders green tea.

Acting, like singing and playing in a band, is in reality an unbeliev-able, spirit-crushing grind. It might be even worse than the music busi-ness. Music you can do on your own. You can play on the street. You can use social media to build an audience. But with acting—unless we are talking about the "acting" that takes place sans clothes for a paying Inter-net audience—you need other people. You need a stage or a camera or, at least, a classroom filled with like-minded colleagues willing to indulge your need to perform. I think almost everyone knows this. It is a fairly accepted reality that acting is a tough way to put food on the table. There are a million jokes that poke fun at how chronically unemployed actors are. (An actor says to his friends at a restaurant: "Good news! I got an-other callback. My agent says it's between me and the guy who's going to get it!") Still, given that one of my goals in this chapter is to inject a bit of cold reality into the subject, and given that tens of thousands of individ-uals hope to use acting as a path—either for themselves or their talented offspring—to celebrity status, it is worth some further exploration.

While we sip our drinks, Ganeshram tells me about the many things he must do to keep his acting career moving: acting lessons, off-off-off Broadway productions, constant hustling, and, naturally, innumerable auditions. One night he performed in front of *one* person—and she was the girlfriend of a cast member. But this is what he loves. At this point, he can't act full-time, which is the norm for most of the people who describe themselves as actors, so he does have a day job. But he is quick to point out that the day job is only to pay the rent. It's not a Plan B. "You can't have a Plan B; otherwise you are going to fail," he explains. He's "all in."

I heard this "no Plan B" theory from another, very successful (i.e., lead in movies and TV shows) actor. The idea is that having a Plan B both compromises your craft and undermines your chance of success. It is as if the success gods are watching and will reward only those who are fully committed. No one deserves entry into the realm of stardom without truly having suffered. "I constantly wonder what else I should be doing. Should I move to LA? Some actors tell me I must move because that is the next logical next step. That is where the jobs are. Others say I should stay in New York because there is too much competition in LA." Ganeshram isn't kidding: there is a lot of competition in Los Angeles. It has been estimated that there are about three times as many actors in that city as there are in New York. Ganeshram is just starting to catch his stride in what I sense is a well-rehearsed rant about the challenges of being an actor in New York when he freezes midsentence.

"Damn! Damn! Where is it?" He suddenly becomes aware that his cell phone is not within earshot. He frantically does the universally familiar cell-phone-search dance. The entire routine is completed within seconds. Front pants pockets. Nope. Back pants pockets. Nope. Shirt pocket. Nope. Jacket. Bingo! And then he stares wide-eyed at the phone. He missed a call. He missed *the* call. "I can't believe it! I've carried this fucking phone with me all day. I even stared at it while I was in the bathroom. I am so sorry. I gotta call them back right now!" He pops out of our booth and executes a quick zigzag exit from the bar, cell phone on his ear.

What are the chances Ganeshram will become a star, which, he had no hesitation admitting, he would "absolutely love, and any actor who says otherwise is a liar"? If we define *star* as a highly paid actor in studio movies, his chances are ridiculously, infinitesimally tiny. Though I couldn't find any hard-core academic research on this point, there are several examinations of the issue in the popular press. For example, the website *Book of Odds* uses the Ulmer Scale (a well-known industry list of Hollywood's hottest actors) to put the chances at an incomprehensibly unlikely 1 in 1.5 million. You have a much better chance of getting killed by an asteroid (about 1 in 700,000). Other, more forgiving calculations take into account that if you are a serious, full-time actor, you really aren't competing against everyone dreaming of being a Hollywood star, just other serious, full-time actors. Still, every calculation I found framed the chances as so remote that if we were talking about an adverse event (such as being struck by lightning) instead of a reaching-for-the-stars ambition (becoming a well-paid actor), we would simply say, *Not going to happen.* True, these kinds of rough calculations are hardly scientifically robust, particularly since, as noted, the denominator includes more than just seriously committed actors. And there is, of course, a huge amount of luck, timing, and genetics (do you look like a movie star?) involved—a point I will return to—that can raise or lower your chances. Just the same, these figures help to convey the rarity of making it "celebrity big" in the acting game.

The statistics related to child actors are slightly more concrete, mostly because the field is somewhat regulated. As a result, more statistics are available, but they're equally gloomy. Each year there are, for example, more than twenty thousand child actors, just counting those with agents, in the Hollywood area alone. If you include *all* the child actors looking for work, the number is likely much larger. I saw one calculation, based on child work permits, that put the number at more than sixty thousand. This city-size horde of aspiring and parentally "encouraged" celebrity wannabes is scrambling for about twenty-five regular TV roles. And a lot of people in the industry, including a former child star, told me that almost all those parts go to kids who already have a significant acting resume. If your child does not already have solid showbiz credits, the chance the kid will get a job is, as succinctly summarized by BizParentz, a foundation dedicated to supporting children in the entertainment industry, "almost zip."

# # #

"SORRY ABOUT THE FRANTIC ARRIVAL. I was just at an audition for some god-awful big budget *roooobot* movie. Even after thirty years, nothing changes. You must audition!"

What's up with actors? It seems that every one I meet is *just* coming from an audition. This robot-movie auditioner is the versatile thespian Michael Simkins. We meet in a charming hotel bar close to Victoria Station in London. Simkins isn't breaking any respectable middle-aged British actor stereotypes. And I mean that in the nicest way possible. He is fun, witty, and articulate. The kind of guy you'd like to have a few pints with. I am thrilled to have the opportunity to chat with Simkins. In acting terms, he has done it all. He has been in successful West End theater productions such as *Chicago* and *Mamma Mia!* He has been in big-budget movies such as *The Iron Lady* and *V Is for Vendetta*. He has been a semi-regular on a TV show, including a recent stint on the popular UK show *EastEnders*. And he has been through the early-career acting grind, which included performing in more than sixty plays in five years. (He can still, from memory, list them all.) Though not quite a celebrity, he is, by almost any measure, a successful working actor. Or, as he puts it, "I am a man who has spent his life somewhere between triumph and complete oblivion." More important for me, he has put a great deal of thought into the challenges of being an actor. He has written two books and numerous op-ed pieces, mostly for the *Guardian*, on his craft. Indeed, for the UK media, he is one of the go-to commentators for all things acting—a status that is confirmed during our discussion by a call from a reporter for meaty actor-ish quotes about some urgent theatrical development.

"Impossible goal. Simply impossible."

This is Simkins's quick response when I ask him if my new friend Ganeshram has a chance of becoming a movie star. I run the better-chance-of-getting-hit-by-an-asteroid factoid by him. "That sounds about right," he says after a pause. "The problem, of course, is that it *does* happen. There are some new actors that make it. Proof that it happens is on TV and in movies. We *see* them succeed. We are dazzled by the possibilities. This allows us to hold on to the dream that we could be the next one. This makes it hard to be realistic."

OK, if we are being realistic, Ramesh Ganeshram has, basically, no measurable chance of becoming a celebrity actor. But what are his chances of becoming a well-paid, regularly employed actor, like the genial man sitting across from me in the London bar is? Though the point here is that using acting as a vehicle to celebrity is folly, it is worth noting that even this far more modest goal is difficult to achieve. It has been said, not coincidentally by Michael Simkins in an op-ed he wrote for the *Guardian*, that actor employment statistics are terrifying, "with something like 92 percent of the profession out of work at any one time." To make matters worse, the same 8 percent tend to get much of the work. So the key is to break into the 8 percent and stay there, always bearing in mind that the vast majority of this 8 percent don't make much money. Life as one of the 8 percent is rarely celebrity posh. As one New York–based actress told me shortly after she auditioned for, but did not get, a substantial role in a Hollywood blockbuster, "Your job as an actor is, basically, rejection and auditioning . . . and more rejection. There is very little actual acting."

BACK IN NEW YORK, I watch Ramesh Ganeshram pace back and forth on the sidewalk just outside the bar while talking on his phone. His body language does not provide any clue about how the audition went. There is no fist pumping or Rocky pose. My guess: no job. Woody Allen famously wrote: "Show business is not so much dog eats dog as dog doesn't return other dog's phone calls." I figure that it is terrific that Ganeshram at least got a chance to audition, and, no matter what news was being conveyed, he has taken another step in the right direction. At least the dog returned his call. I start thinking about the best way to say "too bad" without sounding like a condescending dick.

Ganeshram steps back into the bar. One look at his face tells me my guess was wrong. He got the part. From a selfish point of view, I can't believe my luck. To actually *witness* an actor get a job is a bit like seeing a meteorite hit the ground. You know it happens—the Earth is covered in craters—but to be there when a call arrives seems too good to be true.

"Wow, we shoot on Monday," Ganeshram says with a wide smile. He pushes his green tea aside and orders a beer. "This is a great profession." Time to celebrate. The dream lives on.

Sports Star!

Of course, music and acting are just two of the ways people think about getting famous. Another perceived path to celebrity is through achievement in sports. Indeed, for many young athletes, "going pro" is viewed as an entirely sensible ambition. And, sadly, many parents hold this view as well. In reality, the chance of making it as a sports celebrity, like the chance of making it as an actor, is almost zip. For example, a kid in Canada playing in minor league hockey right now has a much better chance of getting struck by lightning or dying of a flesh-eating disease than of playing a single game in the NHL—even if the kid has been identified as talented, is currently a minor league star, and has all the right support and training. An often-quoted 1999 analysis looked at a group of thirty thousand kids playing junior league hockey in Southern Ontario. Of that number, 235 were drafted into the Ontario Hockey League (the minor league), but only 110 got to play and even fewer, 90, played for more than three years. Of course, the number for those who made it to the NHL—a step necessary in order to have a sports career that would confer celebrity status—was even smaller. Fifty of the thirty thousand were drafted, but only twenty-five played a game. (As it happens, even this number was unusually high—it was a good year.) If you look at the number of players who had something close to what could be called a career—which, in this study, meant players still in the league at age twenty-four—the number drops to just eleven. Bottom line: only eleven out of thirty thousand ended up with a solid NHL career. And that was in 1999. Because there are now more professional players from countries other than Canada, it is even more difficult to break in.

If you want to look at this from a cold statistical standpoint, you *cannot* become rich and famous from professional sports. It is so rare, as is the case with becoming a movie or rock star, it borders on the statistically impossible. Technically, something is statistically impossible only if the chances of its happening are zero, but eleven in thirty thousand is getting darn close to zero. That is 0.037 percent. And comparably grim numbers exist for other sports, such as basketball and football. If you take the high school seniors playing on school teams as the denominator, and generally these are fairly serious athletes, there is only a .03 percent chance of a pro career in basketball. Of 156,000 high school senior basketball players in the United States, only 44 will be drafted to play in the NBA after college. Similarly, there is a .08 percent of a pro career in football. Of 317,000 high school senior football players, approximately 250 get drafted. And it should not be forgotten that "getting drafted" is no guarantee of a career. On the contrary, obscurity is the norm for most draftees.

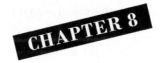

## CHAPTER 8

Celebrity Dreams and Cognitive Biases

Not everyone is pursuing celebrity. When measured against the entire population, the number of individuals who are committed to becoming an actor, singer, or sports star is not huge. One commentator estimated that, in 2009, approximately four million adults in the United States had fame as their primary and explicit goal. Add children and adolescents and that number increases substantially. And, I am guessing, the number likely doesn't include those seeking sports fame, because the goal of becoming a professional athlete is often not characterized as a celebrity ambition. In addition, as the well-known human development scholar Oliver Gilbert Brim noted, "there is an unknown but substantial number of people with the fame motive who deny it to the world and keep it a secret even to themselves." In other words, the pursuit of celebrity may be an unconscious or covert motivator for many people. We may not want to admit it, but the idea of celebrity and fame may nevertheless shape how we think about our goals, activities, and current lot in life.

The belief that fame and celebrity are sensible life options has broad social ramifications. And, while the number of individuals actually committed to chasing fame is comparatively small, it is also not insignificant.

Even if you accept the conservative calculation put forward by Brim, that four million are seeking fame in America alone, this is still a phenomenal number of individuals who will not achieve the celebrity status they so desperately desire and are spending their valuable time on this earth in an utterly futile pursuit.

Indeed, Brim provides yet another example of the massive disconnect between the desire for fame and the actual chance of achieving it. (I promise: this is my last bit of you-ain't-gonna-make-it statistical dream crushing.) Drawing on a number of sources, including the number of hall of fame biographical entries for the fame-related professions, Brim estimated that about twenty thousand "fame slots" are open to the four million fame seekers. (I think this is an overly generous calculation, as not all top-level actors, singers, or even athletes are true celebrities. But supposing he's right, there remain 3,980,000 who are going to be seriously disappointed.) So we know the chances of grabbing the brass ring are slim, and we know that eager hordes keep reaching for it. It is, then, worth considering the cognitive and social forces that keep the celebrity dream alive. Why do so many people believe, despite all the evidence to the contrary, that they're going to be famous? Let's start with what the existing evidence tells us about human nature.

Humans are all, for the most part, wired to be deceived (and perhaps exploited) by the dream of celebrity status. Understanding this cognitive predisposition can help to explain the durability of the search for celebrity, but it also offers insight that, I hope, will help us all to get on with our lives—whether we are seeking to be an *American Idol* finalist or trying to climb the corporate ladder. First off, people are, in general, pretty terrible at assessing their own abilities. College students are bad at guessing their own IQ (usually overestimating it, naturally), and numerous studies have shown that people overrate their creative talents. This has been called, not surprisingly, the "*American Idol* effect." If you have ever watched the show, you have undoubtedly asked yourself, *How in the world does that person think he or she can sing? Is that person completely deluded?* I saw some of them warming up at my audition. Many were truly terrible, but they sang with a bizarre boldness that invited scorn from the other contestants, and they were oblivious of that too. In fact, the kind of squirm-inducing overconfidence that has helped to make shows like *American Idol* entertaining (in that enjoying-the-humiliation-of-others kind of way) may be perfectly natural.

A 2011 study published in the journal *Nature*, for example, suggests that overconfidence and the tendency to overestimate ability is a characteristic conferred on humans by evolution. While this exaggerated confidence can lead to crazy decisions (naked bungee jumping, anyone?) and even put individuals at risk, in the aggregate and over time it has provided us with an evolutionary advantage and thus has established a home in our DNA. The study found, for example, that if the evolutionary rewards (beating a competitor in a fight for food or a fine-looking mate) outweigh the risks (getting pummeled), then being overconfident is, from an evolutionary perspective, a good thing. But the authors of the study note that while overconfidence may have conferred an adaptive advantage in the distant past, it might not be as beneficial in the context of modern society (though it clearly helps the producers of reality TV). Like our evolutionarily determined desire for extra calories—a predisposition that was a big evolutionary advantage ten or twenty thousand years ago—the tendency toward overconfidence might not always work to our advantage now.

The inability to assess our own talent has been found in numerous domains and even among the very young. A study of seventy-eight fourth-grade students, for instance, found that the kids were "remarkably poor predictors of their own creativity." Research on point has consistently found that self-reports about talent—whether in art, writing, science, math, singing, acting, or writing—tell us little about actual, objectively assessed ability. So when Ryan Seacrest asks an *American Idol* contestant about her singing ability and the contestant responds that she is *awesome and that everyone thinks so*, we can be fairly certain that she has no clue—which the show uses to comic effect.

There is a closely related line of studies that have found a strong tendency for people to rate themselves as above average. Indeed, if you believe the evidence, we all think we are pretty darn good at just about everything we do. A well-known 1981 study found that 93 percent of drivers think they are better than average. (From the perspective of my daily bike commute, I'd say that you are *all* seriously and chronically below average. I am, however, an awesome bike rider.) A US study of more than one million high school students found that 70 percent thought they had above average leadership skills. Only 2 percent thought they were below average. Being highly educated apparently does not improve self-knowledge. A whopping 94 percent of university professors think they are above average teachers—which, by the way, I am. Just ask me.

People also believe they are more selfless, kind, and generous than others and, to top it all off, better looking too. Research tells us that most people (particularly men) believe they are more attractive than average. Yes, as I noted earlier, celebrity culture often makes us feel dissatisfied with our appearance or a particular body part. But, for many of us, our built-in cognitive biases also delude us about our appearance. We are, it seems, dissatisfied but still aesthetically above average. Given the role of appearance in the celebrity universe, this is highly relevant to the present discussion. Research by Nicholas Epley and Erin Whitchurch, for example, has found that people are more likely to recognize an attractively enhanced picture of themselves than a less attractive picture (the yep-that-good-looking-person-in-the-picture-is-me phenomenon). Another study, an online survey of more than twenty-six thousand Americans, found that most reckon they're above average in looks, giving themselves a 6 or 7 on a scale of 10. Among those younger than thirty, almost a third think they rank between an 8 and a 10.

While many psychological theories have been put forward to explain our tendency to rank ourselves as above average, recent work by Jonathon Brown from the University of Washington suggests that the primary driver is, quite simply, a desire to feel good about ourselves. In a series of experiments he found that people are particularly likely to rate themselves as better than average on traits that are viewed as socially important, that is, traits associated with character and skill, such as honesty or intelligence. He also found that the tendency increases when people's self-worth is threatened. In one of Brown's experiments he gave half the research participants an intelligence test that resulted in uniformly (fake) low scores. Those who received the insulting results were, when asked about their ability, more likely to rate themselves as better than average compared to a control group that was not similarly insulted. People are predisposed to ignore, or at least downplay, evidence that portrays them in a negative light. But this and other research results also provide insight into what drives people who persist in pursuing celebrity status, namely, their inability to realistically assess their own talent. And when their self-appraisal is challenged by, for example, those cruel *American Idol* judges, their response may be defensive and paradoxical. Instead of taking the advice of the experts and abandoning a singing career, unsuccessful contestants frequently storm out of the audition room, telling the world how great they are and how, one day, they'll be bigger than Michael Jackson.

Not surprisingly, this tendency also applies to how parents view their children. If you go by the perceptions of parents, every kid is above average. Every kid is special, smart, and talented in some unique way. I've got four kids, so I know this tendency well. In fact, my kids seem to be well aware that I lack credibility. I recently effusively praised the baking skills of my oldest daughter, Alison. Alison was unmoved. She looked steadily at me and said: "You are incapable of judging my baking. You are my dad." A good deal of research has shown that Alison is right—though I stand by my assessment of her lemon cake; it *is* first class. Parents aren't terribly good at measuring how their kids stack up. Research has consistently shown that we overestimate our children's abilities in areas such as IQ, memory, and language. An online survey, for example, found that 72 percent thought their kid was smarter than average. Only 6 percent thought their child was less intelligent than average. A 2009 study found that parents overestimated their kids' intelligence even more than the kids did. The study found that teachers were the most accurate predictors of a child's objectively measured intelligence. (Remember this the next time you feel like complaining to a teacher that he doesn't understand your child's unique gifts.) Another study, published in 2013, found that fully 91 percent of parents overestimated their children's emotional comprehension (the important social skill that, among other things, involves the understanding of the nature, cause, and consequences of emotions and the ability to sense the emotional state of others).

In fact, parents aren't particularly adept at evaluating even the basic physical and mental condition of their children. For example, a 2012 US study found that only 15 percent of parents think their kids are overweight, even though research has shown that about 32 percent of kids are overweight or obese. Similarly, parents underestimate the degree to which their children are unhappy or anxious and overestimate the degree to which they feel happy and satisfied.

We're Pollyannas too. In general, we are unrealistically optimistic about the future. This well-established psychological phenomenon, known in the literature as "unrealistic optimism," or "optimistic bias," has been found in innumerable studies. People tend, for example, to downplay the chance that bad things will happen to them. This is one reason why people knowingly do unhealthy and dangerous things. The thinking goes as follows: *Bad things happen to other people, not me! I won't get a nasty disease, so there's no need to wash my hands or quit smoking. I won't put on weight, so I don't need to watch my calorie intake or avoid junk food. And I won't get in a car crash, so there's no need to slow down or wear a seatbelt. I know all those horrid things happen, but they are more likely to happen to someone else.* Note that the cognitive bias of unrealistic optimism also applies to positive outcomes. Most people overestimate the chances that their future will be bright, at least when asked to compare their chances to those of their peers. For example, studies have found that individuals overestimate the possibility of positive financial outcomes, that a cancer treatment will cure them, or that they will achieve particular career goals. Since Neil Weinstein first described it in a famous 1980 experiment, this phenomenon has been demonstrated numerous times. Weinstein's study found that college students rate as better than their peers their chances of, among other things, getting a good job, living past eighty, having an achievement recognized in a newspaper, and getting a career award. While there has been some quibbling in the academic literature since this 1980 study about the strength and source of the optimistic bias tendency, the research to date has been surprisingly consistent. We all think the future will turn out better for us than for the next guy. Again, this has obvious implications for our understanding of the ardor with which some people pursue celebrity status. *My chances of becoming a famous actor, musician, or athlete are darn good, at least compared to yours!* What I find most remarkable, however, is the degree to which optimistic sentiments persist, even when individuals are confronted with conflicting information. Even when they know the statistics that demonstrate how slim their chances are of becoming a celebrity musician, actor, or athlete, they remain immovable. People think the statistics apply to other people but not to them.

In 2011 neuroscientist Tali Sharot and colleagues at University College London published a paper in *Nature Neuroscience* titled, appropriately, "How Unrealistic Optimism Is Maintained in the Face of Reality." Sharot and her colleagues found that the human brain is biologically wired to filter out information that does not confirm previously held optimistic beliefs. Sharot's team studied both the brain (using a special MRI machine) and behavior of research participants as they dealt with information that confirmed or conflicted with a previously held optimistic picture of the future. What they found was that humans selectively update knowledge and beliefs in a way that makes unrealistic optimism extremely resistant to change. Our brains let in and process the stuff that seems to support our unrealistic views while seeking to keep out all the negativity. As Sharot and her colleagues conclude: "Our brains and behavioral tendencies make us peculiarly susceptible to view the future through rose-colored glasses."

There are many specific examples of the operation of these biologically affixed rose-colored glasses in ways that directly support my supposition that they play an important role in the continuing desire to achieve celebrity status. I corresponded with Sharot on this point and she agreed, saying the evidence tells us "people will continue believing in their dreams, even when faced with information that suggests it might not be a good idea."

An early paper with a particular focus on celebrity-oriented professions came to the same conclusion as Sharot. Those engaged in "artistic professions," the authors suggest, "are [the] most likely to succumb to this particular kind of over optimism." The authors note, for example, that girls training to be ballet dancers persist in their belief that they could have a professional career "even if explicitly confronted with the cruel facts, in particular that the rate of unemployment is extremely high and the income low." They found that the "girls dutifully listen to such information, [but] they are unshaken in their overoptimism believing that this may well be true but applies to the others." The authors also conclude that the same overestimation applies to would-be actors; the researchers cast acting as "one of the professions with the highest rate of unemployment in the whole labor force."

Studies also have shown that the optimistic tendency plays out in sports. A 2012 study from Germany, for example, followed almost sixteen hundred elite-level soccer players aged ten to twenty-three. The players all attended the training academies of the thirty-six German Bundesliga (the top tier) professional clubs. These academies are the primary source of professional soccer talent in Germany. So being asked to participate in one of these academies is a big deal—a sign you have true soccer talent. A majority of the players thought their chances of becoming a star were good. This belief endured even though it is well known that the chances of success are slim, even among this assemblage of tremendously talented and handpicked youths. How slim? Fewer than 5 percent will sign a professional contract, let alone have a significant, celebrity-worthy career. And yet, even though these young men could actually *witness* the rarity of success as they watched the vast majority of their older colleagues fail, they clung to their belief in their own glorious destiny. Indeed, the trend toward unrealistic optimism was remarkably strong in every age group. Even the older players in this study believed, on average, that their chances at success were good. This result surprised even the lead author of the soccer study, Verena Jung, from the Institute for Sports, Business, and Society at EBS University in Germany. "I expected that the older they become, the more they would get realistic about the judgment of their chances," she told me. "But I found the opposite to be true."

The huge social profile of celebrities, the celebrity-making process, and celebrity lifestyle add to the power of these cognitive biases. Celebrities are everywhere in popular culture, so it is not hard to find an example of a person who has "made it" by following a path similar to the path *you* are struggling on. I spoke to one actress who is no longer young by Hollywood standards (though she *is* young if measured against a normal standard for humans) and who continues to get a reasonable amount of work. She told me she remained hopeful about her chance for big success. As proof she pointed to several actors who made it late in life. "I am on my own path," she told me, "but just look at these other actresses who made it late in life! I know it can happen." Success stories exist that illustrate the possibility of triumph over almost every type of adversity. If you want to be a professional athlete but never got drafted by a professional team, you can turn to many examples for inspiration and "evidence"— albeit anecdotal in nature—that success is still possible. The future Hall of Fame quarterback Kurt Warner, for example, was never drafted and had a job packing groceries before he landed a job with an NFL team. Now he is considered one of the best quarterbacks of all time. If you are no longer a teenager and still crave success as a pop star, you can look to Sheryl Crow—she was a near-ancient thirty-one years old when she first made it big. And if you do not conform to the Hollywood stereotype of beauty and thinness, you can point to full-figured actresses like Melissa McCarthy and Queen Latifah.

The tendency to seek out and use information that confirms previously held beliefs is called confirmation bias and is, of course, closely related to the neurological and behavioral phenomenon I just described. Much has been written about this tendency in the context of politics. Conservatives see and seek out evidence that confirms their conservative beliefs, whether it is about gun control, taxation, or gay marriage. Liberals do the same. When it comes to the topic of climate change, it has been demonstrated that individuals gravitate toward "evidence" that supports their worldview—no matter how crazy or marginal. Confirmation bias can affect personal decisions. And, I believe it plays a particularly salient role in why fame and celebrity are viewed as obtainable and desirable goals, either by individuals in relation to their own career choice or by parents in relation to their kids. Stories of success have huge sway. Indeed, research has shown that a single powerful anecdote can have more persuasive force than a mountain of statistics, and this seems particularly to be the case in the context of celebrities. Their stories of success fill magazines and other media, and when they are presented from the perspective of a wealthy actor, singer, or athlete who is looking back on life, they can appear to be compelling proof that a celebrity life is not that far out of reach.

Sunk Costs and No Plan B

Many of the people with whom I spoke were neither naive nor young. On the contrary, many had been at the fame game for a long time. I spoke to actresses and actors in their midthirties and to full-time touring musicians who were well past the age at which many people are married and have families. They seemed to be well aware of the odds against their achieving real success and money. Nevertheless, they stuck with it. Why? Of course, many of them simply love the life and the artistic process. But numerous other forces add to the pressure to continue following your dream.

For example, research tells us the longer people stay in the game and appear to be taking steps toward success—not getting cut from a sports team, getting a callback for an acting job, performing at SXSW—the more likely they'll hang in. On some level, this may seem like a logical decision: after all, these aspiring stars are receiving positive feedback that suggests their chances at success are increasing. But to believe this is to forget that the longer they pursue a dream job with a low chance of success, the more the opportunity costs increase—in terms of money, time, and future career options. That is, as one gets older (and for most of the fame-game professions, that is the midtwenties), the risks intensify. So even if the chances of success go up (e.g., you've made it to a high-level sports team or gotten a small part on a TV show), so do the costs. One would think that this reality would cause people to reevaluate. But another cognitive bias, often called the tendency to honor sunk costs or the escalation of commitment, can kick in, making a career adjustment difficult.

Cognitive bias applies even if we aren't succeeding at our chosen career. It happens even if, from an objective point of view, it appears that we are failing to achieve our stated goals. This is because the more we invest in a decision, whether in terms of money or time, the more likely we are to find ways to justify and rationalize the decision. It happens with gamblers (hold instead of fold). It happens with investors (buy instead of sell). It happens with married couples (counseling instead of divorce). And it happens with prime ministers and presidents (um . . . war in Iraq).

I asked the TV and movie actor Bryan Greenberg about the Plan B mentality. I wanted his view for two reasons. First, he has had a terrific career, with leads (e.g., *Prime*) and great parts (e.g., *Friends with Benefits*) in many Hollywood movies and starring roles in successful TV shows (e.g., *One Tree Hill* and *How to Make It in America*). I think it fair to say that he has achieved celebrity status. Second, and more important, he is the guy who gave my new friend Ramesh Ganeshram the no–Plan B advice. "The reason I never had a plan B when pursuing my dreams is 2 fold," Greenberg told me in an e-mail. "One: I wasn't good at anything else. And two: The path to success in my field is so challenging that I knew if I gave myself an out, I would take it. Humans always take the path of least resistance. So I just put side blinders on and trotted down one path."

This strategy seems nearly suicidal, at least from a life-plan perspective. I asked Michael Simkins about it during our discussion in London. "Only an actor would understand this," he said. "It makes total sense. If you have a Plan B, it can easily become Plan A. You get used to the security and to the money associated with a real job. Suddenly Plan B is Plan A, and, before you know it, you aren't acting anymore. If you get off the acting tightrope, it is hard to get back on." From the outside, those caught in the vortex of an escalation of commitment often seem irrational. But you can see how it can happen. When you have invested time, money, and effort in a particular activity, it can be very difficult to walk away or cut your losses, even if, from an objective point of view, that is the more rational decision.

The trap caused by the escalation of commitment catches parents too. Increasingly, kids focus on one or two activities at a young age. The costs and time investment can be significant. Hockey parents in Canada, for example, invest thousands of dollars on sticks, skates, power skating lessons, hockey camps, travel, and the like. The authors of a recent book, *Selling the Dream*, found that it isn't unusual for families to sink more than $300,000 in a youngster's hockey career (imagine if they had invested that money!). Parents may feel that, given this commitment, they should keep going, even if Junior isn't looking like the next Wayne Gretzky.

A friend and colleague, Camilla Knight, studies the role of parents in the experiences of child and adolescent athletes. Before her life as a researcher, Knight was an elite tennis player. So it is no surprise that much of her research has focused on tennis parents. During her academic career—Knight is now a lecturer in sports psychology at the UK's Swansea University—she has interviewed hundreds of parents. She has found that the motivations for putting kids into a particular sport are of course complex and varied, but that many parents do hope their child's participation will lead to a successful collegiate or professional career. "If they stop funding or supporting their children in the way they have previously," Knight told me when I asked her about the problem of escalating commitment, "parents can feel that all their previous support has been for nothing. . . . In fact, one parent best described it to me as being like a hamster on a wheel and not being able to stop."

She told me about another aspect of the sunk-cost dilemma, one that is unique to parental support. "Having committed so much already, they find themselves in a difficult situation because they feel that suddenly stopping could prevent their children from succeeding . . . or be viewed by their children as an indication that their parents no longer believe in them."

SO WE ARE biologically and cognitively set up to believe the celebrity life is both realistic and attainable. We are terrible at assessing our own abilities. We are neurologically constructed to be unrealistically optimistic about our future. We have a tendency to seek and use information that confirms our beliefs and to ignore facts that conflict with those beliefs. And once we are on a particular career path, we may find it difficult to cut our losses. Adding to this near-perfect storm of cognitive tendencies is that most of us are appallingly bad at comprehending probabilities. Indeed, we are not good, in general, at thinking statistically, particularly when the relevant probabilities are extremely remote. If the numerator is exciting and well publicized and the denominator huge, we have a tendency to focus on the numerator. This relates to another common bias called denominator neglect. When we hear, for example, that only eleven out of thirty thousand minor league hockey players will play in the NHL, the numbers have little persuasive force because—again, for most people—they just don't mean anything. People see the success of the few, well-publicized sports stars, and this guides their perceptions of chance. Many parents likely think: *Hey, eleven kids made it!* Or: *Well, my kid could be one of the eleven; I like them odds!*

Not long ago the *Winnipeg Free Press* carried a story about the vast amount of money that hockey parents invest in the sport. A few sentences uttered by one of the parents interviewed by the reporter serves as a powerful example of how long odds can be known but still not resonate. "I'll guarantee you one thing," the hockey dad said. "If you don't buy a lottery ticket, you can't win. That's why, if parents can afford it, they will pay. . . . Everybody says only one player will make it out of a million. Why can't it be yours?"

Of course, in this context, the lottery ticket is not a piece of paper purchased at a corner store but a child's time, a family's resources, and, perhaps for all of them, lost opportunities to experience other things.

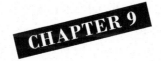

Simon Cowell and
Social Pressure

"You can sing," Simon Cowell told Rachel Miller after she finished a jazzy version of "Somewhere Over the Rainbow." Cowell's praise was delivered in his now infamously snide and matter-of-fact tone. To the then-seventeen-year-old Miller, it didn't feel like much of a compliment. "I thought he was being sarcastic!" she told me with a laugh as she reflected, eleven years later, on her *American Idol* experience.

Though she always dreamed of being a famous actor, she was often told she had a good voice and not just by family members. So when the auditions for the first season of *American Idol* rolled through Chicago, a short trip from her hometown of Madison, Wisconsin, she was encouraged by family and friends to give it a try. *American Idol* had not yet become the cultural phenomenon we know today, and she saw participation as a bit of a lark and an opportunity to get more singing experience. At that point in her life she had already committed a lot of time and energy to acting and singing, mostly in musical theater. Fame and fortune were the objective. "I am from a lower-middle-class family. The fantasy, the ultimate goal, was high income. [Stardom] is portrayed like you will get millions."

Miller also told me that she felt a lot of pressure—from family and from society generally—to follow her dreams and reach for the stars. To never give up. To strive for fame. To be her best. To never say never. These were the messages she got from everyone in her social sphere. "Not that it's bad or that I didn't appreciate the support from family and friends," she told me. "But all of the cards I got were 'Follow your dream' cards."

I have discussed the powerful individual psychological, and even evolutionary, predispositions that keep the celebrity dream alive. But, as Miller's comments highlight, there are also social and economic forces at play. This includes the Western world's love affair with ambition and the idea of "following your dreams." This love affair is relatively new. For most of human history ambition was viewed as either a vice or a sin. (For example, Shakespeare warned us in *Henry VIII*: "I charge thee, fling away ambition: By that sin fell the angels.") But during the past hundred years or so, the mix of consumer culture and the rise of the American dream ethos recast ambition as a virtue. It is tough to escape the reach-for-the-stars mentality. It is everywhere. Using an Internet search tool (Google Books Ngram Corpus, which gauges the frequency with which a phrase appears in the millions of English-language books published over decades and yields an indication of linguistic and cultural trends), I traced the incidence of a range of phrases associated with chasing our celebrity dreams. What did I find? Since the mid-1950s we have been increasingly bombarded with phrases that tell us to never give up, to dream big, and to reach for the stars. In fact, virtually every phrase that I could think of as an analog to the idea that we should "follow our dreams" has increased in use since 1950. That key phrase has increased in use by a factor of about fifty. In other words, it is used fifty times more often now than it was in 1950. (To be honest, the phrase was almost *never* used in the 1950s, so my calculation is conservative.) "Never give up" has increased in use by a factor of 6.2; "reach for the stars" by a factor of 27; "dream big" by a factor of 21; "believe in yourself" by a factor of 8.9; "never say never" by a factor of 54; "be your best" by a factor of 4.3; and "do not give up" by a factor of 3.7. In contrast, consider these words and terms that have *decreased* in frequency since the mid-1950s: *sacrifice*, *appreciation, obligation, service, teacher, engineer, fine arts, public interest, public duty,* and *economic equality.*

Research by Yalda Uhls at UCLA found a similar trend when she analyzed the most popular TV shows aimed at teenagers. She set out to map the degree to which, among other things, the value of "fame seeking" was embraced by the main characters. The results are striking. Fame seeking went from fifteenth place (last place on the list of values analyzed in the study) in 1967 to *first place* in 2007. The study, published in 2011, also found that the value of "achievement" rose from tenth place in 1967 to second in 2007, and the value of "community" fell from number one in 1967 to eleventh place in 2007.

Of course, the relationship between popular culture and social values is complex. The media both reflect and shape popular perceptions. But whether the popular representations I mentioned earlier are leading or reflecting public sentiment, it is hard to deny that a shift has occurred. In our current culture, the idea of bettering ourselves and seeking fame is framed as a noble endeavor, almost a social expectation. If you have a chance to make it celebrity big, that should be your central priority. Just think of all the heart-wrenching story lines from shows like *American Idol, The Voice,* or *So You Think You Can Dance,* where a contestant must put individual dreams of fame over, say, staying with a dying parent or working at a job to put food on the table for a young family. The sacrifice for the (illusory) ticket to fame is presented (usually over a bit of sentimental pop music and with the requisite tears and hugs) as the right and honorable choice. The sacrifice for a shot at fame is what is expected of you.

(Quick side observation regarding *So You Think You Can Dance:* This is an entertaining show but wealthy celebrity dancer? You have a better chance of being abducted by aliens and crowned the ruling monarch of Alpha Centauri.)

Rachel Miller's *Idol*-propelled search for fame continued past the audition phase, though she soon would make a curious, and culturally antithetical, decision about her career. After a brief round of banter among the *Idol* judges, Paula Abdul announced, in a bubbly Paula Abdul manner, that Miller had made it through to the next round. "Work on your stage presence" was Cowell's last bit of advice, halfheartedly lobbed in Miller's direction as she was heading out of the room. At least that is how she remembers the otherworldly encounter. Months later, she found herself in "Hollywood" (in the first year of *Idol*, the famous "Hollywood week" actually took place in Pasadena) for the next round. She didn't last long. Once again, the judges thought her stage presence was not *Idol*-esque. She got the boot.

She told me the *Idol* experience was fun, a great opportunity and just as weird as you might expect. "Everyone was very nice, and, yep, many of the contestants were there solely because they wanted to be famous," she said. But she wasn't overly concerned about not progressing. She had other plans, including competing at an event in New York sponsored by the International Modeling and Talent Association (IMTA).

IMTA IS THE largest modeling and performance association in the world. It has also been called the most expensive. Participants in the IMTA convention can pay as much as $10,000 for an experience that is portrayed, mostly by IMTA, as a stepping-stone to superstardom. These conventions are attended mainly by kids, teenagers, and young adults desperate for fame and celebrity. And the organizers play to this constituency. IMTA, according to its website, "is the place where the world's top model and talent agents, managers and casting directors come to find new faces." It is also, for the vast majority, the place where young wannabe celebrities are separated from a significant amount of money for the privilege of, basically, hanging out with, and competing against, other wannabes.

The existence of entities like IMTA highlights the other force driving our social commitment to the celebrity dream: fostering and supporting the dream is a massive and profitable business. The celebrity industry, which includes dance classes, singing lessons, modeling conventions, online "talent agencies," and beauty pageants, exploits the fantasy of celebrity and all the cognitive predispositions and personal vulnerabilities that keep the fantasy alive. Indeed, from the perspective of this industry, the more the prospect of celebrity seems to be a tangible and reachable goal, the better. The industry has nothing to gain by telling aspirants to celebrity the truth.

A significant portion of fame-oriented competitions, classes, and services seem to be full-on scams. Do not let yourself or (more likely) your kids succumb. A modeling class, for example, cannot teach you to be tall, beautiful, photogenic, and rail thin. That requires, in descending order of importance, genetics, genetics, genetics, and, if genetics don't do it, a diet of water and lettuce. An open audition for a kid show that sounds too good to be true *is* too good to be true. These are swindles designed to hook families into spending ridiculous amounts of money for photos, representation, acting classes, and so forth on the promise of a chance to appear on TV. The Disney Channel is often rolled out as a potential employer. Real TV shows don't need to hold open auditions in malls to find actors.

Unlike most of these exploitative ventures, IMTA conventions appear to have helped a few current celebrities to achieve success. Indeed, what makes IMTA conventions alluring is that many well-known actors and models are alumni/ae of these events, including Ashton Kutcher, Katie Holmes, Jessica Biel, and Eva Longoria. Many of these stars give glowing testimonials on the IMTA website. Holmes, for example, gushes thus: "Let's just say, a girl from Toledo would never end up in a Hollywood movie if it weren't for the IMTA." (That kind of analysis of a personal career trajectory is undoubtedly distorted by another cognitive bias called hindsight bias. It is likely that when Holmes looks back through the lens of a successful—albeit a Tom Cruise–tainted—career, it seems to her that IMTA played a significant role. Her assessment doesn't, obviously, include the sizable role played by luck. Nor does it include consideration of the thousands upon thousands of wannabes who took the same steps and never got even a nibble of interest.) While there are a handful of IMTA alumni/ae who have made it celebrity big—a fact that IMTA deploys to create a glamorous narrative to overwhelm the grim statistical reality— it is easy to find stories of heartbreak associated with participation in the IMTA conventions. An article in the *New York Observer* describes a young woman who lost more than $42,000 in her efforts to achieve celebrity through IMTA. "I didn't have tons of money beforehand, but the agency just told me to charge it to credit cards and that I would make it all back within a year when I was famous," she told the magazine.

I thought I should check out IMTA myself, but no one from the organization returned any of my e-mails. So I dropped by the conference uninvited.

The New York event is held in a large hotel in midtown Manhattan. As soon as I walk in the front door, I see gaggles of young, attractive model types. I am clearly in the right place. Moments later, a half-dozen shirtless, well-built, twentysomething, unself-conscious men zip by, in a hurry to get to a place where shirtless men are urgently needed. I meander around the lobby chatting with participants. I meet a thirteen-year-old from Chicago ("I can act, sing, and dance!"), a twenty-year-old from South Africa ("I hope to be a successful model"), two teenage boys from Canada ("we always wanted to be famous"), and a seven-year-old who wants to be like Selena Gomez. It goes on and on. When I ask why they came to the IMTA event, almost all say they view it as a stepping-stone to stardom— often seeming to paraphrase IMTA promotional material—and several drop references to Katie Holmes as evidence to support their decision (confirmation bias in action!). The seven-year-old used a crowd-sourcing website to raise the money necessary to attend IMTA. (I was told by most that the cost was about five thousand dollars, but no one would give me an exact figure.) The child's website informs contributors that she needs to get to IMTA because it is a "once in a lifetime experience" and her "biggest dream would ultimately to be an actor with Disney Channel."

Numerous seminars are under way. I stroll down a hallway and stick my head in an open door. At the front of the hall sit two bored-looking men (I later find out they are moderately successful casting directors). The room is full of children and parents. There is a long queue of kids behind a microphone anxiously waiting their turn to ask the two men for advice. They all ask some version of the same question: How do I become famous? And the answer is always the same: Work hard, prepare, and make the most of every opportunity. Just before I turn to leave, a little blonde girl, who looks to be about seven or eight, gets on her tippy toes and asks, "How do you make a casting director remember you?"

One of the men smiles, leans into the microphone, and says, "Well, darling, just be as cute as you are now." Sage advice.

A section of the conference floor is roped off. This is the competition area. It is the main ballroom and where the bulk of the participants seem to be located. I try several times to talk my way in. No luck. Finally, after a long chat with one of the conference "guards" (he looks more like a model than a bouncer) to explain my project, I get escorted inside. The area is set up like a fashion show, with a well-lit runway and large video screens on either side. As I walk in, grade-school boys are, one at a time, working the catwalk in the "jeans competition." An announcer with a voice that has a beauty-pageant vibe calls out a four-digit number ("neeeext up . . . five-threeee-nine-siiiiiiiix!"), and a small boy wearing the designated number confidently marches down the runway with all the swagger of a high-end model who has done it a million times before.

I am standing behind the panel of judges, who seem only half interested. They will grade the little models, and a few boys—very few—will get a callback and the chance to do it again in front of agents, casting directors, and their ilk. I have absolutely no idea what the boys are being graded on. How does one nine-year-old wear his jeans better than the next nine-year-old?

BUT WHAT ABOUT our *Idol* castoff, Rachel Miller—how did IMTA treat her? Was the convention in New York an expensive, fruitless scramble for a grab-and-a-miss at the celebrity brass ring?

In fact, Miller's experience at the IMTA event turned out to be the kind of anomaly that keeps the illusion of fame alive. Like the participants with whom I spoke, she paid big. She told me that though she can't remember details, she believes her participation in the event cost about $2,500, plus airfare and hotel. She also needed to pay for professional photos in order to produce a model-quality portfolio. This cost more than $1,000. For a family without a lot of money, this was a significant investment. But, amazingly, her participation in the event *did* result in the promised meetings with well-established agents. She won or did well in all the IMTA competitions she entered, including the singing and modeling categories. And this led to a contract with a respected talent agency with offices in New York and LA. Next up for Miller was a move to LA and work with a hit-generating music producer who has written or produced songs for the likes of Celine Dion, Kylie Minogue, and Eminem. Miller's dreams of fame and fortune nudged significantly closer. *This is really going to happen*, the seventeen-year-old thought. *I am going to be a star.*

Please Note: Punctuality Is Extremely Important!

If you spend any amount of time online researching the concept of celebrity, one thing quickly becomes clear: a lot of companies are ready to help you become famous. There are, for example, StarNow ("where talent gets discovered . . . actors, models, musicians wanted . . . no experience required"!), Casting Now ("a platform to showcase your talents"), Click-MyTalent ("a talent profile service"), and One Source Talent (OST). The last one is ubiquitous. Indeed, many other online celebrity career services funnel you back to OST. A well-known modeling company called Model Search America—a company that says it will "see you at the top"—has an "apply now" link after the question "Do you want to be a model or an actor?" The "apply now" link takes you to One Source Talent. The exact function of OST is unclear, but the flashy website, which prominently displays the company's tagline—"No more what ifs"—makes it appear that a career as a model or actor is both common and easily obtained. On the home page is a picture of a teenage girl (most of these celebrity-focused companies seem to be aimed at tweens and teenagers) with "Become a Model/Actor" written next to her smiling face.

Sounds good! I decide to sign up.

I click on the "apply" link. This takes me to a registration page that starts with the question "Are you ready to take your shot?" In addition to my views on "shot taking," they want my name, date of birth, e-mail address, and phone number. That's it. I also upload a picture of my old, less-than-celebrity-like face. I push the "submit" button and, no exaggeration here, I *instantaneously* get a call. I swear the call came so fast that I had to lift my hand from the mouse to my cell phone, which told me a call was coming from New York.

"Um . . . hello?"

"Hi! This is One Source Talent!"

"Wow! You guys are fast. No fooling around!" I respond.

"Well, you know what this is call is about!" replies the friendly and enthusiastic-sounding woman. "We are having an assessment here in New York in a few days. Would love for you to come by."

I agree that it sounds like a great opportunity, even though I have no idea what an assessment is.

More than anything, these online services (I use that term loosely) appear to be a way to exploit the desire for a glamorous career by promising to get you exposure with casting directors and modeling agents. These companies refer to a range of jobs in the entertainment industry, though their connection to these jobs is unclear. It seems likely they simply want their clients to believe there is a link and that there are, in fact, thousands of jobs available. The Model Search America website, for example, says that there are "all kinds of opportunities out there" with "the millions of TV networks" that "need content to fill air time." This remarkable claim is followed a few sentences later by this: there "are thousands of networks out there too" (what happened to the millions?), including "Disney, Fox, CBS, NBC, ABC, ESPN, VH1, MTV, FX, Comedy Central, Discovery Channel, Food Network, Spike, TNT, Spout, Nick Jr., E Entertainment and the list goes on and on." The webpage concludes thus: "If you want to be on these networks you have to start somewhere and that is why Model Search America is here for you."

"I'm looking forward to my meeting," I tell Jennie, my new personal contact at One Source Talent. She tells me that I don't need to bring anything to the assessment. No special clothes. No prepared bit of acting that someone can use to "assess." And no special photos or acting resume. But, I suspect, a credit card might be needed.

I decide to get my assessment at One Source Talent's Hollywood office. That way, when I get signed to work on a big studio movie, I won't have far to go. A few days before my appointment, I get an e-mail from OST. I am told to "dress to impress." That "punctuality is extremely important. Do not just be on time; be early!" And to "relax, be yourself and professional. When your opportunity comes to shine, stand out with a positive attitude and professional behavior."

I arrive at OST early. How could I not? An attractive young receptionist in the slick-looking office greets me. A framed magazine cover behind her tells me that OST was, in 2008, one of the country's fastest-growing companies. There are about twenty people in the room with appointments at the same time as mine. Most are young children with their parents. The latter primp and fuss over their aspiring little celebs: there is much anxious pacing, hair spraying, combing, and parental injunctions to "stand up straight." It all got me a bit nervous. Perhaps I was a tad unprepared. A young man wearing a bowler hat (and a smile that, I think, had a wisp of irony attached to its edges) called out my name and invited me to get in a line for a picture, which, another pretty young woman told me, was "purely for our records." Beside me was a boy who appeared to be about five years old. He was wearing a flashy outfit that looked like a little version of a tux you might have worn on a Vegas stage circa 1970. His name was Sparkle. "Just Sparkle," he said confidently to one of the OST staff. (He actually had a different, but similar, one-name name.) Sparkle was called in for his assessment before I was. As he disappeared into an office, I heard a female voice say something like, "Hi, Sparkle, I am the head of West Coast youth talent identification." About ten minutes later it was my turn. Pretty young woman number three invites me into a small office. She tells me to stand in front of her desk for the "audition." Not an assessment but an audition. Gulp. *Are they going to ask me to act?*

"So what are your career ambitions?" she asks.

"Nothing too grand. I am always looking for new experiences," I reply ambiguously.

"Do you have any experience?"

"Actually, I was the lead singer for a rock band," I say, keeping it truthful but leaving out any reference to the relevant decade.

She then asks me about my day job ("I have flexible hours"), whether I would be ready to work soon ("Sure!"), and whether I have professional photos. I respond with a yes to this question; I had them done for my last book. She informs me that I will probably need new ones, even though she has no idea what my old ones look like.

"Well, you have a great look." I do not. "You are perfect for something we have coming up next week," she says. "Be ready for a call! Thanks and good-bye."

That was it. No singing. No acting. No posing. I interacted with OTS staff for a total of about two minutes, and that included asking pretty young woman number one to order me a taxi. I didn't have much of an opportunity to shine, stand out, or display my positive attitude and professional behavior.

I wonder how much time Sparkle got.

MONTHS PASS AND I never get the call. Apparently, my look isn't *that* great. I do, however, continue to receive regular e-mails from One Source Talent asking me to come in for an assessment. Clearly, I did not shine or stand out enough for them to remember that I have already had one.

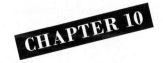

Luck and Ten Thousand Hours

"One thing people don't understand is that there is so much luck involved." This reality dawned on Rachel Miller after just a few weeks in LA. "I am not a great singer," she told me with a laugh. "I'm good. But I got lucky. Luck got me to LA. There are so many talented girls. So many! I was in the right place at the right time. You need so much luck to get anywhere."

Luck plays a significant role in every career, of course. The adage about being in the right place at the right time could apply to almost any profession, from accounting and teaching to playing quarterback for the New England Patriots. ("Dear Drew Bledsoe, Thank you for getting injured. Love, Tom Brady.") But because of the huge number of people scrambling for a small number of fame-creating positions, and because the public, casting directors, music producers, and the market all are fickle, luck plays a particularly significant role in the realm of celebrity. Also, unlike, say, being a track-and-field champion, success at a celebrity job depends on a great deal of subjective assessment—an assessment that can be influenced by a boatload of uncontrollable factors (did the casting director have enough coffee before you walked into the room?). As of this writing, Usain Bolt is the fastest man alive. Period. Who is the best actor or singer or even quarterback? (OK, the last one is obviously Tom Brady, but some may disagree. They would be wrong, but other, less informed opinions exist.)

Many actors and musicians I spoke with, especially those who had enjoyed a degree of success, shared Rachel Miller's appreciation of the massive role of luck. Michael Simkins put it this way: "Luck is more important than talent. Theoretically, you can get by without talent. Talentless actors make it. But without luck, you are fucked." This view is also held by the stratospherically successful, or at least that is what I have been told by a reliable source. Tim Monich is a renowned acting coach. He taught at Juilliard in New York for years and now works closely with the biggest stars on planet Earth, including Brad Pitt, Tom Cruise, Leonardo DiCaprio, Cate Blanchett, Nicole Kidman, Matt Damon, Clive Owen, and Juliette Binoche, to name but a few. Monich was in Vancouver working with Owen and Binoche when he and I met up in a downtown coffee shop. He told me emphatically that all the stars he works with—*all*—realize how lucky they are. "Leo and Brad? [*Leo* and *Brad* . . . love it.] Yes, they are ridiculously good looking and talented. They work very hard. But they *know* how lucky they are. All are very aware that they have won the lottery."

The philosopher Seneca said, "Luck is what happens when preparation meets opportunity." This saying, a go-to axiom for motivational speakers, football coaches, advice columnists, and inspirational kitty posters, is, with all due respect to the dead Roman, wrong. Luck happens to those who are lucky. Period. And, please remember, the distribution of luck is random. That is why it is called luck. You can't do anything to enhance your luck.

Despite the honest calculation of the role played by luck in the careers of the artists I interviewed, a calculation that apparently resonates with seriously lucky Leo and Brad, many of us often greatly overestimate the degree to which we can control the uncontrollable. We imagine, for example, that our thoughts and actions can have an impact on outcomes that are entirely or largely beyond our control. This phenomenon, known as the illusion of control, operates in a range of contexts, including gambling, investing, and the management of health risks. And like many of the other related psychological traits (unrealistic optimism, overconfidence, optimistic bias), maintaining this illusion seems to have a biological foundation, a proposition confirmed by recent brain-scan research. This is because appreciating causal connections—seeing a relationship between actions and getting food or avoiding a predator, for example—conferred an evolutionary advantage. As such, we err on the side of seeing a connection, even when there isn't one. And because we see a connection between a particular action and a particular outcome, we think our actions can have tangible impact. We are, in short, wired to believe we can control the uncontrollable.

Adding to this illusion is the widespread belief that celebrities have, to some degree, earned their status. It wasn't luck but skill and hard work that led to their fame and fortune. The survey of 650 American teenagers cited in a previous chapter, for example, asked teenagers to consider why celebrities became successful. The respondents selected "hard work" more often than all the other options combined, including luck and innate talent. Why is this relevant? Even though we are constantly told "If we can dream it, then we can achieve it," dreaming and achievement are, in fact, usually only tenuously connected. It is an illusion that one leads directly to the other. The talent pool is so massive and the assessment criteria are so complex and ambiguous, to say nothing of such factors as timing and genetics, that landing a celebrity job is probably 90 percent luck. Yes, for many jobs, particularly in the sports realm, you need to have the requisite talent and training to hold a ticket in the lottery, but luck still looms large. To paraphrase the Nobel Prize–winning psychologist Daniel Kahneman, career success is the result of talent plus luck. Great success (i.e., celebrity-size success) is the result of a wee bit more talent and an incomprehensible amount of luck.

The point here is that you can't, through hard work, practice, or positive thinking create the luck or circumstances that will vault you to celebrity status. In the realm of music, for example, bands that have little hard work–enhanced musical proficiency populate the lists of the best bands in history (e.g., the Ramones and, my personal favorite, the Clash). And there is at least some evidence that the quality of a song has little to do with whether it will be a hit. In addition to the roles of marketing and timing, an element of randomness is involved in determining what becomes popular. In a 2008 study, the sociologists Matthew Salganik and Duncan Watts found that perceptions of success seem to influence purchasing decisions more than quality. They created a list of songs and allowed approximately thirty thousand individuals to download their favorites, which resulted in a ranked list. The sociologists then inverted the list, so that the least popular songs now were ranked as the most popular, and invited another group to download their favorites. As the authors had predicted, the songs deemed unpopular in the first round were now popular. Although some of the "best" songs rebounded, a clear self-fulfilling-prophecy effect was at work. Songs viewed as popular become popular. In other words, the cream does not always rise to the top. Momentum, which the authors call "cumulative advantage," and luck rule.

I am not arguing that talent and hard work are irrelevant. On the contrary, for most celebrity jobs, you need both simply to enter the lottery. Talent and hard work are often—but not always—the minimum prerequisites. I am suggesting that, for most celebrity-oriented careers, you also need a huge amount of luck, a factor that is totally out of your control. Realizing this injects an important reality check into the discussion. You can't plan on and work toward being lucky. And you can't plan on or work toward becoming a celebrity. To suggest otherwise, as implied by our society's obsession with the idea of reaching for the stars, is to promulgate a lie.

THINK I AM being too harsh? J. K. Rowling stands as another great illustration of the degree to which luck plays a role in the context of celebrity professions or, really, *any* profession. She has sold approximately 450 million books, making her one of the best-selling authors in human history. The eight Harry Potter movies are, according to some estimates, the largest-grossing film franchise ever. Now, given this status, and her millions of admiring fans, surely it was hard work and raw talent that propelled her to fame? Doubtful. Once again, luck had to be involved. And Rowling provides us with a bit of evidence.

In 2013 she wrote a crime novel, *The Cuckoo's Calling*, under a pseudonym, Robert Galbraith. The result? Some publishers turned it down. One of these now-red-faced publishers has since acknowledged that she thought the manuscript was not particularly original, lacked a clear selling point, and "didn't stand out." When it finally did get published, it received solid reviews, but sold fewer than five hundred copies. Keep in mind that Rowling already had a literary agent, which is one of the first and biggest hurdles in the writing world. If she didn't have an agent, the manuscript might not even have been considered for publication. My guess is it never would have been published at all.

When it was revealed that Rowling was the author, the book instantly became a best seller, making this rare real-world experiment an illustration of the random nature of success. Duncan Watts, one of the authors of the song study I mentioned earlier, commented that the Rowling book controversy demonstrated "that quality and success are even more unrelated than we found in our experiment." And "it is also clear that being good, or even excellent, isn't enough."

BUT WHAT ABOUT sports celebrities? Success in the domain of sports isn't haphazard or arbitrary. The most talented and hardworking succeed. Right?

In fact, research tells us that, for most sports, success appears to be the result of a relatively random process that is, once again, influenced by luck and other factors that are out of our control. Some "measurable" performance-oriented sports, such as, say, sprinting, depend less on luck and rather more on talent, but luck is still involved. The element of luck begins with the genetic characteristics your parents "decide" to provide. And then your genetic gifts must be recognized and nurtured. After all, there may be someone out there who's even faster than Usain Bolt but doesn't know what he's got. As for the big professional sports—football, baseball, hockey, soccer, and so on—it is shockingly difficult to predict who is going to succeed. Even if an NHL team drafts a player—in itself a rare occurrence—the odds are that the draftee will not play in the NHL. Ditto for the NFL. And if you don't get picked up relatively soon after the draft process is over, the chance of ever getting picked up diminishes rapidly.

There is evidence of this kind of randomness in other sports too. For NFL quarterbacks—an absolutely *massive* financial investment for the owner of a team, so you know that the quarterback-assessment experts are doing everything within their power to get the selection process right—a careful historical analysis found that the relationship between actual performance and draft position is weak. Despite analyzing mountains of player performance data, dissecting hours of video of quarterback candidates, and watching quarterbacks run through a range of assessment exercises and considering the tens of millions of dollars that are at stake, experts still don't know how to predict success. Indeed, studies have found that outside the first-draft round, the relationship between how high a player is drafted and actual playing time is not particularly strong. This is true for all the major professional team sports. Athletes drafted in the first round do play more frequently than others, at least initially, but that may be due more to concerns about "sunk costs" than actual talent. That is to say, teams may tend to play the guys in whom they've invested the most cash.

These findings about the rather arbitrary nature of the draft system and the difficulty of measuring and predicting success in professional sports are important from the perspective of this book because they highlight the somewhat ad hoc nature of making it as a professional athlete. Obviously, you must possess otherworldly physical talent even to be in the mix. But you also must be the right player, in the right place, at the right time. In other words, even if you are handed the perfect genes and have the best parental and coaching support, an obsessive drive, and an incredible work ethic, making it as a professional athlete greatly depends on blind luck.

# # #

THOUGH BEING REALLY good at something—singing, playing guitar, dancing, acting, hockey, football—is absolutely no guarantee of fame and fortune, the question remains: How does a person become celebrity great at something? Can you work and dream and "never say never" your way to greatness in preparation for a run at fame?

Malcolm Gladwell's best-selling book *Outliers* made the ten-thousand-hours rule famous. The premise is that almost anyone can achieve greatness at an activity—golf, tennis, chess, violin, guitar—if they put in enough time. And "enough time," or so Gladwell's theory goes, is ten thousand hours. This jibes with the idea that hard work, persistence, and following your dream will inevitably lead to success. It provides us with a sense of control over our future and a way to combat the notion that all is not, in fact, luck and innate talent.

It's an interesting theory, and it appeals to my egalitarian sensibilities. But the data are far from conclusive and, I think it is fair to say, suggest that the ten-thousand-hour theory is, at best, only part of the story. Indeed, for some activities, particularly in the area of sports, it is obviously wrong or at least incomplete. I could train for twenty thousand hours and never run a fast marathon or be a great pitcher or a world-class golfer. A great deal of sports aptitude is dependent on innate ability largely determined by your biological, and particularly your genetic, makeup. A 2012 study published in the *British Journal of Sports Medicine* sought to tease out the relative contributions of genes and training in the development of an athlete. The authors conclude: "Although deliberate training and other environmental factors are critical for elite performance, they cannot by themselves produce an elite athlete." For that, you need a whole bunch of luck in the genetic lottery.

But what about such pursuits as music, which appear to be less constrained by physical abilities? (Acting and modeling also are, to a large degree, constrained by your gene-determined looks, so I'd put these two celebrity activities in the same category as sports.) Can a musician practice her way to greatness? Not likely. Research by Zach Hambrick and colleagues explored the degree to which the amount of practice predicted the ranking of musicians. They found that practice accounted for 30 percent of the variance in the rankings. In the conclusion to their 2013 paper, they write: "Deliberate practice is not sufficient to explain individual differences in performance." Thus more than two-thirds of an individual's ranking as a musician is determined by factors other than practice—and, more than anything, that other stuff is probably innate ability.

"Many want to believe that if you are sufficiently motivated, any-one can become an expert at something," Hambrick, a professor of psychology at Michigan State University, told me. "But the data simply does not support this position." He feels that the ten-thousand-hours idea endures because it fits so well with both democratic ideals and the anyone-can-make-it ethos of the American dream. It fits with the dream of celebrity. "While it may be a nice idea," Hambrick says, "it just isn't true." Or, as perfectly encapsulated in the headline for an article he wrote for the *New York Times*: "Sorry Strivers, Talent Matters."

I am not a genetic determinist. I do not, for example, think that we will be able to develop a test that will inform wannabes whether they have the right genetic makeup for a particular celebrity profession. The roles played by genes and human behavior are just too complex. Nor do I think we should let our genes constrain or dictate our future. If you are a short, slow man and want to play point guard, go for it. But know that ten thousand hours of hard work will not overcome the short, slow stuff. I have played guitar for more than ten thousand hours, probably closer to fifteen thousand. Seriously. I love it. And I am brutal. Terrible. I seem to be incapable of improving. It is as if I were stuck in a rut of mediocrity. Most of us are. That's why it is called mediocrity.

Even Sir Paul McCartney, whose success Gladwell explicitly attributes to the ten thousand-hours rule, questions the theory. "I mean there are a lot of bands that were out in Hamburg who put in 10,000 hours and didn't make it, so it's not a cast-iron theory," McCartney said. He thinks that most groups that are successful put in a huge amount of work, but, he says, "I don't think it's a rule that if you do that amount of work, you're going to be as successful as the Beatles." Indeed. And the reverse is also true. Many successful bands had far fewer than ten thousand hours behind them when they signed a contract. As noted, many bands have been signed despite a lack of musical proficiency. It is often said that U2, one of the most successful bands in rock history, started writing songs because they couldn't play covers well enough.

It is obvious that the genetic lottery, and many other forces outside our control, combine to create innate ability. They all have a huge impact on our chances of fame-generating greatness. And this is just another way that luck reigns over our celebrity aspirations.

Lucky Rachel

So how did luck play out for Rachel Miller? Did it propel her to a celebrity career? In fact, luck did quite the opposite, and she couldn't be happier.

Before she left for Los Angeles, she applied to and was accepted by the University of Wisconsin. But at that point in her young life, she was still committed to a career in the entertainment industry, so college was a backup plan (yep, her Plan B). Still, she thought it couldn't hurt to attend the freshman orientation event before she made her big move to the West Coast. Seated across from her in a huge university hall, as the usually gregarious Miller explains, was "the first man I couldn't talk to. I was totally tongue-tied." As luck would have it, that man was her future husband.

Her experience in LA played out as one might expect, though it was hardly glamorous. She moved into a small place with another young woman who was also seeking fame and fortune. Miller met regularly with her producer and other musicians to write and strategize. And she was pushed to change her look. Many, for example, told the modeling-contest winner that she needed to lose a few pounds—and her name. At the time, the pop-punk star Avril Lavigne was big. Scrambling to find the "it" factor by capitalizing on the Avril wave, it was (pathetically) suggested that her new name should have some of the same Avril edge. The moniker "Madison Tyler"—the first name was a reference to her hometown—was selected. Naturally, she would also be expected to change her sound to fit the name. No jazzy interpretations for Madison Tyler.

She was offered a contract, but the whole thing didn't feel right to her. "I would have been creating a pop album for money and fame," she said. "Those are the wrong reasons." She felt this way even though fame and fortune had been the whole point for her, from a young age. But when she saw the contract laid out in front of her, it no longer seemed attractive. And, perhaps most important, she couldn't stop thinking about that man. "So I told them thanks but no thanks," Miller told me. "They looked shocked. I don't think they had ever had someone turn down a contract."

She headed home to Wisconsin. She got great marks and became the first person in her family to graduate from college. She went to law school. She became a lawyer for the federal government. And, of course, she got married to that man. Many of her friends didn't, and still don't, understand her decision. "Even my parents," Miller tells me, "bless their hearts, because they were incredibly supportive during this whole process, were frustrated that I walked away." Everyone kept asking her why she would give up on her dream. You aren't supposed to stop reaching for the stars, especially when they are within your grasp. But that isn't her view. "Saying no to that contract was the best decision I ever made." Not a hint of regret.

Miller has never sung professionally since that time. Occasionally, she will do some karaoke. "It is fun to shock people!" she told me with a laugh. One night in 2008 she did just that. On a whim, she jumped on stage to sing karaoke in front of a local band. A reporter caught the performance and was impressed. He noted that the "slim, pretty Rachel" would "look good on a CD cover" and might be just the kind of singer that could catapult the band "into international superstardom."

Reality TV and YouTube

Many individuals, including people in the entertainment business, suggested to me that it was now easy to become famous because of social media and reality TV shows. This may *seem* to be true. There are a lot of these shows around. And they offer a way to move rapidly up the fame food chain. During my travels and research for this book, it seemed as though I heard the name Kim Kardashian almost every day. She certainly shows up in *People* a lot; she was in nearly every issue I read for a year.

But the impression is misleading. It is still incredibly rare, as *American Idol* contestants can attest, for individuals to become celebrity big through reality TV. While I could not find any systematically collected statistics, the number of individuals who have gained big-time celebrity through a reality show remains small. Indeed, one could argue that the phenomenon of reality TV, with its emphasis on the desirability of stardom, has drawn more individuals into the fame-seeking game, thus increasing the denominator and, as a result, making true celebrity status even more unlikely. The number of people playing the lottery has increased.

The same can be said of YouTube. Sure, many individuals have gained notoriety (OK, a select few have become *huge*, such as Justin Bieber), and some have used it to build on an existing career (e.g., Psy with the hit "Gangnam Style"). But few have built a career solely through YouTube to the point where they have broad name recognition and substantial wealth. This is starting to change. For those younger than twenty, You-Tubers, as they are often called, have become increasingly well-known personalities. Still, how many YouTube celebrities can you name, not including Bieber and Grumpy Cat? Then think of the tens of thousands of videos that exist. Do the math. You can make money from YouTube (advertising revenue is shared), but unless you get millions of views, the income is insignificant—between eighty cents and six dollars for one thousand views. With approximately one hundred hours of content being uploaded *each minute*, the chance of standing out is astronomically slim. Again, though quality plays a role, luck is obviously a big, big factor.

I am not denying the rising power of social media or the way they can facilitate the creation of artistic communities or even satisfy elements of the desire for fame. Much has been written, for example, about the rise of the "microcelebrity," individuals who build and play to a relatively small audience. But in the search for mainstream, big-time celebrity status, YouTube, and, for that matter, Facebook, Instagram, and Twitter, have emerged more as an expected part of a wannabe's reach-for-the-stars portfolio than primary vehicles. They are powerful tools, but that's all.

And, as with reality TV, social media increase the number of individuals seeking celebrity—expanding the already enormous denominator—by making it easier for more and more to play the fame game.

Another theme I heard expressed involved the conflation of fame, success, and talent. Indeed, the actor Olivia Munn picks it as her number-one issue. "The worst part about fame," she says, "is that some people confuse fame for success." What she and others are concerned about is the ability of social media and reality TV to propel people to a kind of talent-free fame. "But just because people want your picture or know your name, doesn't mean you have success," Munn says.

"Andy Warhol would have loved it," the long-time publicist Susan Blond tells me of the current wave of people who are famous for simply being famous. "Kim Kardashian? Warhol would have loved her. She's fun. She's kitsch." Blond should know. She worked with Warhol. She also worked with the Clash. The first thing I notice in her New York office is a framed gold record for the Clash's seminal album, *London Calling*, my all-time favorite. Seeing it there gave me goose bumps. Blond was in several of Warhol's films, including the black comedy *Bad*, in which her character throws a screaming baby out the window. The scene is still hard to watch. She also worked with Britney Spears and Ozzy Osbourne. Blond is just as engaging, opinionated, and fun as you would hope some-one with her eclectic background in the entertainment industry to be. She inspired the character of the publicist Bobbi Flekman in the movie *This Is Spinal Tap* ("Money talks, and bullshit walks!") but has none of her edge. Thank goodness.

"Well, you might say they earned it. Some had sex on video" is her joking response when I ask if reality stars have earned their celebrity sta-tus. Blond seems to view the famous-for-being-famous phenomenon more as an element of popular culture than as some kind of irritatingly unjust achievement. As Bobbi Flekman might say, It's all bullshit—why split hairs? "To be honest, it is hard not to be jealous of the people who have figured how to make money off of just their celebrity status. They get paid a huge amount just to go to parties," Blond says. Paris Hilton reportedly made about half a million for simply showing up at events.

This phenomenon has helped to promote the idea that fame, and not the fostering of exceptional artistic talent, is a reasonable goal all on its own. This is why, I suppose, some kids say they want to be famous and not, for example, a great guitar player or an exceptional actor.

Blond is quick to dismiss those in the industry who claim to be above the drive for celebrity status. "Make no mistake: many great artists love the idea of fame. And I like celebrity. I like fame," Blond says. "But I get more excited about raw talent."

So What?

In this section of the book, I have touched on a few of the myriad reasons it is nearly impossible achieve true celebrity. In many ways, our entire social economy creates a massive pop-culture-fueled positive feedback loop that builds the illusion that celebrity status is both an attainable and a reasonable goal. And this illusion is kept alive by, and plays to, our biologically determined cognitive biases, which make us all susceptible to the belief that we can—and should—"reach for the stars" and "never say never." You may be thinking, so what? What does it matter that the illusion of celebrity-size success shapes the hopes and ambitions of kids, families, and struggling artists and many others besides? The answer is simple. If we can see through the illusion, then we can make more in-formed decisions. And being aware of our cognitive biases allows us to be more sensitive to our actual strengths and weaknesses. This awareness will, I hope, allow us all to avoid celebrity-dream scams. Potentially, it will keep us from committing large amounts of personal and family resources to an unattainable goal. This is both a philosophical issue (do we really want a society in which celebrity status is a primary goal?) and a practical challenge with real consequences. For example, a 2008 study of UK teachers revealed a growing concern about the impact of celeb-rity culture on the education environment because, as one teacher said, "pupils believe celebrity status is available to everyone" and students "do not think it is important to be actively engaged in school work as edu-cation is not needed for a celebrity status." Another noted that students "believe that they are much more likely to achieve financial well-being through celebrity."

More broadly, it should give us pause that so much of the modern world's social capital—in terms of time, cultural space, and economic investment—is geared toward selling and seeking a goal that is, for all practical purposes, nonexistent. The American dream is based on the idea that if you work hard enough, you can have a good life and do whatever you want. But the whatever-you-want carrot that is meant to drive our society forward does not—again, in any real sense—exist. The carrot at the end of the stick isn't real.

On a more personal level, the realization that the chance of making it celebrity big is so remote, and so dependent on factors that are completely out of our control, is liberating. Accepting that frees us from the constraints and economic pressures involved in trying to "make it" as a rock star, movie star, or sports star. It allows those of us with a passion for sports, acting, or music to embrace the activity for its inherent pleasures and rewards. Many of the people I interviewed, such as Michael Simkins, seem to have embraced this approach from the start or at least came to it at some point in their career. My friend and SXSW tour guide, C. J. Murdoch, is fully aware that he will never make buckets of money or achieve fame in the world of music. Despite this, he made exactly the opposite decision that Rachel Miller made. He turned his back on a successful legal career to live the life of a working musician. "When I started down this path," Murdoch told me, "I took a hard look at the things I have to give up to commit to a career in an area where uncertainty is lord: owning a house, getting married, having kids. I'm prepared to not have any of those things."

His picture of his austere future life is a long way from the "big bucks," "big mansion," "living the high life" celebrity aspirations disclosed in the public perception research I cited at the start of this chapter. But why would Murdoch make such a commitment? As he told me while we watched one of his friends perform on a tiny, unofficial SXSW stage, "I do it because I love it. I love the lifestyle. I love being on the road. And I love making music." In other words, it makes him happy.

#   #   #

WHEN I RETURNED home from my trip to New York, my kids were intrigued by my discussions with struggling actors and musicians. The
Caulfield family loves pop culture. I told them about Ramesh Ganeshram and the breakthrough audition that led to his winning a spot on
Law and Order. When the date of that episode arrived, I watched with
my cop-show-loving daughter, Alison. About forty-five minutes into the
show, during a scene in a hospital, Ganeshram appeared on-screen—for
about ten seconds. He opened a door, approached a woman in a hospital
bed, handed her a paper, and said his one line, "You've been served!"

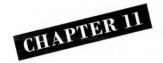

CHAPTER 11

A Lonely,
Health-Destroying Grind?

So obtaining a celebrity job is so rare that it borders on the impossible. Nevertheless, nabbing one is widely perceived as a reasonable, and obtainable, goal. Indeed, pursuing rock star, sports star, or movie star fame seems often to be cast as a noble pursuit ("reach for the stars!"), albeit one that can consume a significant amount of time and financial resources. This raises another interesting question, why would anyone want to be a celebrity? Sure, there are many individuals working in the entertainment industry who are happy and fulfilled, just as there are in any sector of society. But if you believe the research and, for that matter, many of the stories featured in the celebrity media, being a bona fide celebrity seems to be about as rewarding as a prison sentence. And a bit of research backs this proposition.

Studies consistently show that being in a solid relationship is good for you. Research tells us it benefits our mental health and stress levels and is linked to living a long life. A 2006 paper in the *Journal of Health and Social Behavior* went so far as to suggest that "the evidence linking social relationships to health and mortality is as strong as that linking cigarette smoking, blood pressure, and obesity to health." A 2010 review of the evidence, published in *PLoS Medicine* came to a similar conclusion, suggesting that the "influence of social relationships on the risk of death are comparable with well-established risk factors for mortality such as smoking and alcohol consumption and exceed the influence of other risk factors such as physical inactivity and obesity." Other studies have consistently shown that marriage, in particular, is good for health. And this is especially true for us men (likely because we can barely take care of ourselves). Evidence from large cohort studies—big studies that follow large groups of individuals for a long period—have found that married men have a 46 percent lower rate of premature death than unmarried men.

So, in terms of well-being and health, relationships, particularly with a significant other, matter. They matter a lot. But, as everyone on planet Earth (and every assiduous reader of *People*) likely knows, being a celebrity is tough on relationships. The divorce rate among celebrities is much higher than the already-grim divorce stats for the general public, which hovers at 40 to 50 percent. Some estimates put the divorce rate for professional athletes somewhere between 60 and 80 percent. And I have had bouts of the stomach flu that have lasted longer than some celebrity marriages. (Britney Spears and her childhood friend Jason Alexander were married for just fifty-five hours.) In fact, celebrity divorces are so predictable that they are, um, entirely predictable.

In 2006, *New York Times* columnist and social psychologist John Tierney and science writer Garth Sundem came up with a formula for forecasting the duration of celebrity marriages. It considers such variables as age, the relative fame of the husband and wife, their marital history (i.e., how many divorces are already on the books), and the degree to which they are regarded as sex symbols. This formula successfully predicted the breakup of Demi Moore and Ashton Kutcher, Pamela Anderson and Kid Rock, and Britney Spears and Kevin Federline, among others. As succinctly summarized by Tierney in a follow-up article published in 2012: "Fame, as measured by Google hits, is no good for a marriage."

Of course, there are many other hazards to being a celebrity, including the not insignificant fact that it might cause you to die before your time. A much-publicized study, "Dying to Be Famous," published in 2012, compared the mortality rate of 1,489 rock and pop stars to that of the general, nonfamous public. While the relationship between fame and mortality varied depending on the characteristics of performers—solo careers appear to be particularly risky—the study found that, in general, "mortality increases relative to the general population with time since fame." A similar 2007 study looked into the life expectancy of more than one thousand musicians involved in the top one thousand albums of all time. "From 3 to 25 years post fame, both North American and European pop stars experience significantly higher mortality (more than 1.7 times) than demographically matched populations in the USA and UK, respectively." Yet another study, published in 2013, looked at mortality across all the fame-oriented professions, including acting, sports, music, singing, and dance. The authors, who examined one thousand obituaries in the *New York Times*, found that individuals in celebrity-oriented professions died at a younger age. They concluded: "Fame and achievement in performance-related careers may be earned at the cost of a shorter life expectancy."

To be fair, there are a few studies on the other side of the health-risks-of-celebrity debate. Some research suggests that a higher social rank causes animals, including humans, to live longer. Similarly, a 2008 study found that winning a Nobel Prize increases the longevity of a winner, at least compared to that of an individual who was merely nominated, by one to two years. Some speculate that the status from the award gives winners a degree of psychological resiliency that allows them to handle stress better, and, as a result, they live longer. However, a much more modest "social rank" effect was found in other research that is closer to the world of actual celebrities. (I doubt most Nobel Prize winners experience the same substance abuse, relationship instability, and privacy pressures encountered by, say, Justin Bieber.) A 2011 study of actors who win an Academy Award found little evidence to suggest that the status they gained conferred significant life-extending benefits.

In total, while it is tough to do quality research on the issue, and only a few less-than-methodologically-ideal studies are on point, it seems fair to conclude that fame isn't all that good for your health. The increased mortality is likely the result of a combination of factors, including the lack of solid relationships and the embrace of risky and health-destroying behaviors (smoking, drinking, drugs, crazy diets). However, some have speculated that the stress associated with the pressure to achieve and sustain celebrity status could also be a contributing factor. Richard Epstein, an oncologist and coauthor of the obituary study mentioned earlier, has pointed to the destructive effect of the psychological and family pressures that favor high public achievement. An interviewer for the Australian Broadcasting Corporation asked him if the take-home message from this research was *don't aspire to be famous*. His response: "I think that's what I'd tell my children. I think I'd be very worried if my children were too fixated on achieving stardom."

Still, the rich and famous are, at least, famous and rich. Their lives may be slightly shorter, but at least they have lots of money, right? In fact, things look pretty depressing in this domain too. Even if you are lucky enough to make buckets of money through some celebrity-oriented profession, history tells us that the wealth may not last. There have been so many high-profile celebrity bankruptcies that it almost seems the norm. Consider this list of stars who have gone broke: MC Hammer, Larry King, Burt Reynolds, Willie Nelson, Mike Tyson, child actor (and once the highest-paid on TV) Gary Coleman, singer Toni Braxton (twice!), Grammy winner Lauryn Hill, and football great and ten-time Pro Bowler Lawrence Taylor. Celebrity bankruptcies are so common that they may have altered the public's attitude toward bankruptcy. Rafael Efrat, a business professor, has argued that by publicizing celebrities' bankruptcy filings, "the media may have shaped public perception on the subject, making the traditional bankruptcy stigma less pronounced."

Just how often do celebrities get into financial trouble? Though I could find no scientific examination of the percentage of celebrities who go broke, a bit of data available from the sports world gives a sense of how rare financial stability can be for the famous. A 2009 *Sports Illustrated* investigation into the finances of professional athletes reported that 78 percent of former NFL players have "gone bankrupt or are under financial stress because of joblessness or divorce" and that within five years of retirement, an estimated 60 percent of former NBA players are broke. Since the length of a professional athlete's career is extremely short—in the NFL, for example, the average is somewhere between three and six years, depending on how you count—these are likely young men, many without marketable skills beyond their athletic abilities. (And remember how vanishingly rare it is to become successful enough in any celebrity profession to make money that you can then lose.)

So maybe being a celebrity is not all it's cracked up to be. In fact, a few actual studies have tested this proposition. One, published in 2009, involved in-depth and prolonged interviews with fifteen high-profile celebrities, including individuals from the worlds of acting, music, and sports. The authors' goal was to get a sense of what it is like to be famous. What are the advantages and disadvantages? The celebrities were not named, but I can report, after chatting with one of the authors, that they were authentically successful and well known. Naturally, the celebrities listed the expected benefits, such as material wealth (which, as noted, is not always sustained), privileged access (again, temporary, unless celebrity status continues), and a feeling of symbolic immortality. But the interviewees also disclosed many significant downsides, including loss of privacy, feelings of isolation, the inability to trust others, and the need to create a "character-split" between the celebrity entity and the private self. This split can cause significant personal challenges. As Elvis Presley observed: "The image is one thing and the human being is another. It's very hard to live up to an image, put it that way." The celebrities complained about the need to always "be on," that "you are an animal in a cage," that "being a famous person is a full-time job" (something I also heard numerous times while I was doing this research). Overall, you certainly don't get the sense that these celebrities were exceptionally happy or that they felt as though they lived in Shangri-La or had found the pot of gold at the end of the rainbow. On the contrary, the authors note, many report a "sense of loneliness at the center of the fanfare of fame."

"This remains one of the only studies on how celebrities truly feel about being famous. But given how important the concept of celebrity is to our society, we need more work on the topic," Donna Rockwell, the lead author, tells me. Rockwell is a clinical psychologist. Prior to doing her PhD, she worked in the celebrity universe as a TV journalist and producer, and this background gave her access to the celebrities she interviewed. I tell her that my general impression is that there is a sadness that permeates what she heard from celebrities. "Yes, there is an unrelenting darkness there," Rockwell says. "The isolation, the lack of trust and the loss of privacy wears on them. . . . Celebrity life often leaves them feeling empty and broken."

These issues are bad enough for those who are at the peak of their celebrity, but for those whose fame-enhanced status has lost its luster, the psychological issues can be even worse. It is no fun being a former celebrity. For the no-longer famous, it's often all downside (loss of privacy, isolation) and no upside (money, privileged access). Many former stars spend the rest of their lives being asked, "Didn't you used to be . . . ?" The implication, of course, is that they aren't someone now. Rockwell reports in her article that one subject in her study was the lead in one of the "greatest singing groups of her time." While her name is still known around the globe, she is now broke and struggles from day to day. "It is really heartbreaking," Rockwell says.

Rockwell cautions that we need to be careful not to generalize the results of her study too broadly; after all, she interviewed only fifteen celebrities. Undoubtedly some feel happy, fulfilled, rich, and, well, on-top-of-the-world fabulous. Still, her work provides valuable insight into the harsh realities that can accompany celebrity life. It also raises interesting questions about why so many want to be a celebrity. "Anyone who has fame and celebrity as a goal needs to see a psychiatrist," Rockwell says only half jokingly. "It really makes no rational sense."

The Little House of Hedonic Adaptation

All the women in my house love *Little House on the Prairie*. They love the books, the TV show, and the entire *Little House* gestalt. My oldest daughter has dressed up as the main character, Laura Ingalls, for Halloween. Twice. So has my wife, Joanne. My poor parenting skills are often compared to the unflappable, ever capable, and deeply caring approach of the *Little House* patriarch, Charles "Pa" Ingalls—as in: "I don't think Pa would have handled it [fight/upset child/milking of a cow] that way" or "Pa could probably fix it [plugged toilet/leaky roof/broken promise due to airing of important NFL game]." And power outages are viewed as a terrific opportunity to live life "Ingalls style."

As a result, my status on the home front rose considerably when I announced that I would be interviewing Alison Arngrim, the actor who played Laura Ingalls's nemesis, the spoiled and conniving Nellie Oleson. The character of Nellie, with her curly blonde hair (a very expensive wig, it turns out) and stuck-up nose, was a central part of the *Little House* narrative. As a general rule, everyone who loves the show despises Nellie. To do otherwise would be akin to cheering for Snidely Whiplash to defeat Dudley Do Right or for Darth Vader to lure Luke to the dark side. Indeed, as revealed in *Confessions of a Prairie Bitch*, Arngrim's wonderful 2010 autobiography, the first review she received about her acting had more than a dash of venom. Arngrim was twelve. The review was delivered in a loud, clear voice by a classmate hanging out a second-story window during a school recess break: *"You biiiiitchhh!!!"*

"There are many who still think of me that way," Arngrim tells me. "People approach me in restaurants to let me know! Some of it is tongue in cheek, some of it is not."

For those too young to remember the show, some history and context are likely in order. *Little House on the Prairie*, which aired from 1974 to 1983, followed the life of a nineteenth-century American farm family. It was tremendously popular. The Nellie Oleson character was so cruel to the sweet and always kind Laura Ingalls that Nellie quickly became an icon of evil, so much so that *Vanity Fair* once declared Nellie Oleson the number-one female villain in TV history. Syndication of the show—it has run in more than 140 countries—has allowed the Nellie aversion to live on. *Little House* is *still* shown on numerous channels throughout the world.

Arngrim meets me in a well-known bar in the heart of West Hollywood. As we chat, a few patrons stop by to say they are fans. Just as

Arngrim starts telling me about the enduring loathing people harbor for Nellie, a woman, as if on cue, points at Arngrim and says: "I used to hate you." Arngrim smiles, waves, and says thanks. No edge or bitterness. She comes across as friendly, warm, and genuine—one of those immediately likable people. This is Nellie Oleson? Nope.

"Why would anyone want to be famous? It is not that much fun," Arngrim tells me. And she should know. Not only did *Little House* make her famous, but she grew up in the midst of famous people. Her parents were involved in the entertainment business, and her brother was also a successful child actor. At one point her family lived in the Chateau Marmont, a Hollywood hotel with a celebrity-rich history that includes famous deaths (John Belushi died of a drug overdose in a hotel bungalow), injuries (Jim Morrison, who briefly lived in the hotel, fell off a balcony), romantic encounters (Clark Gable and Jean Harlow), and, of course, epic parties. For a good part of her life, Arngrim literally lived in a celebrity-filled world. It was her norm.

But Arngrim also spent many years struggling with the costs of fame, the challenge of trying to transition into stardom as an adult (this included roles on shows like *The Love Boat* and *Fantasy Island* that were calculated to be provocative), and then life as a "former star." She has an intimate knowledge of both the celebrity world and the impact of the various shades of fame on one's life.

SO WHY DO people want to be famous? As I've described, there are many possible explanations, including a range of hardwired cognitive biases and the peculiar pressure exerted by popular culture. But what are people *seeking* in celebrity life? And why don't the harsh realities of celebrity existence dissuade more? My review of the research exploring this issue highlights several relatively obvious themes, including a desire for wealth, a luxurious lifestyle, attention, admiration, status, and the sense that celebrity will grant a degree of symbolic immortality. In his book, *Look at Me: The Fame Motive from Childhood to Death*, Orville Gilbert Brim speculates that the desire for fame flows from the basic human need for acceptance and approval and that it is intensified in some children because of less-than-ideal relationships early in life. It is, in other words, a built-in desire that, for some, is intensified by life circumstances. "The fame motive will not go away but must be endured as a kind of chronic hunger," Brim writes, "never completely satisfied for the rest of one's life."

While Brim's depiction may seem a bit grim and hyperbolic (a chronic hunger?), some recent empirical work supports his view. A study published in 2013 used an online survey to explore the personality tendencies that are associated with the appeal of fame. The authors found that higher "belongingness needs"—that is, a strong desire to feel accepted and included—were associated with an increased interest in all aspects of fame (e.g., having status, being well known and highly visible, and having the ability to support family and friends). It isn't necessary for me to go into too much detail about the psychological traits of individuals who have a strong or near pathological desire for fame (though I will talk about narcissism in a moment); readers will agree, I think, that this social trend is gaining strength. That said, research suggests that the desire for fame is associated with a number of identifiable personality characteristics, including a particular vulnerability and desire to make one's life better. A 2010 study by John Maltby, for example, found, among other relevant personality traits, "an interest in fame emerging as a desire to overcome negative feelings" and a lack of confidence that leads to a desire "to escape aspects of their current life or character by becoming famous." John Gountas at Murdoch University surveyed more than five hundred individuals for a study published in 2012. A clear theme of materialism emerged: simply put, some people want to be famous to get the tangible benefits of fame. Celebrity status, he reported, is seen as "a vehicle for the achievement of a particular lifestyle that satisfies personal goals." Gountas subsequently commented that he was motivated to do the work because he believes the increasing desire for fame is "not just a blip on our radar, but actually a large social and cultural change among young people."

It seems to me that these findings go to the heart of the illusion that achieving fame and celebrity will confer certain benefits and will, ultimately, make us happy, which, we now know, is far from a certain outcome. As Marilyn Monroe once said of fame, "It's like caviar, you know—it's good to have caviar but not when you have it every meal every day."

Like Monroe, Arngrim does not see fame or celebrity as an avenue to happiness or self-improvement—on the contrary. "Being famous is hard," she says after reflecting on the struggles of Justin Bieber, Cory Monteith, Mischa Barton, Paris Jackson, and other young celebrities. "It should never be the goal. If you are unhappy, getting famous is the biggest mistake. Fame doesn't fix problems; it amplifies them. Gasoline on a flame. A small problem becomes a gigantic one." To support this bleak assessment, Arngrim points to the numerous celebrity suicides and suicide attempts. I could find no definitive scientific data to back up her speculation, but some media reports have suggested that celebrities, particularly those who have acquired fame as a result of appearing on reality TV, commit suicide at a higher rate than the general public. While there is, obviously, a causation issue (is it celebrity life that is the problem or does the prospect of celebrity attract individuals who are more likely to be psychologically fragile?), we can say with a degree of certainty, I think, that there is little evidence, anecdotal or otherwise, to support the notion that fame will help to resolve psychological issues.

One study, published in 2013, examined the circumstances attending the suicide of seventy-two celebrities. Using biographies as source material, the authors found that in 97 percent of the cases, there existed a tension between individuals' aspiration for success and the reality of their situation—at the time of their death, the celebrities wanted to be more successful than they were. The authors hypothesize that this strain may contribute to the risk of suicide. They also note that celebrities are, in general, unusually ambitious, and consequently it should be no surprise that their aspirations outstrip objective assessments of their chance of success—a point I've touched on throughout this book.

Suicide is a tremendously complex phenomenon with causations that are, as a psychiatrist I know observed, idiosyncratic and personal. We should take care not to overinterpret the conclusions from this study. Still, the research raises intriguing questions about the psychological impact of our society's love affair with a celebrity-oriented, reach-for-the-stars kind of ambition, especially given the illusory nature of both the goal and the chance of success.

AT THIS POINT, you might be thinking that all this negativity sounds like sour grapes. I failed at my lame attempts at rock 'n' roll glory, so now I am trying to rationalize my mundane existence. This is a logical—and probably not entirely inaccurate—assessment. Also, as noted, some celebrities are perfectly content. So, in order to provide a bit of balance, it is fair to consider the genuine advantages of fame. With this in mind, I searched the popular press for any celebrity quote that described the perks of fame. This approach, I admit, was far from methodologically rigorous. The celebrities could be lying, the quote could be from a publicist, and many of them come from sources such as *People*, which is hardly a repository of deep thinking. Still, I did find a pretty consistent, and oddly food-oriented, theme.

Most celebrities acknowledge that they love the special treatment and day-to-day conveniences afforded by fame. Who wouldn't? As Woody Allen said recently: "You get better seats at the basketball game, and you get better tables and reservations [at] places, and if I call a doctor on Saturday morning I can get him." The actor Chris O'Donnell (*Batman and Robin*, *The Scent of a Woman*, and *NCIS: Los Angeles*) said, "The best thing about being famous is getting a nice table at a restaurant." Kelly Clarkson also likes having the ability to drop her name to get restaurant reservations. Apparently she has an assistant do the name-dropping. "I've never dropped it myself though. I'd feel like a tool." (Yes, Kelly, having your personal assistant drop your name is much less tool-ish than doing it yourself.) Jennifer Lawrence, who has said that fame has ruined her personal life, likes the little things, such as being able to take stuff from the minibar in her hotel room. The actor Jessica Chastain (*Zero Dark Thirty*, *The Help*) appreciates the access to and opportunity to wear designer clothes. Britney Spears says, "The cool thing about being famous is traveling. I have always wanted to travel across seas, like to Canada and stuff." (Real quote. Not the best example, admittedly, but I just couldn't resist.) Even the *Twilight* star Robert Pattinson, who has had few good things to say about fame, admits he likes "staying in fancy hotels with incredibly nice bathrooms."

Another big draw, and, I suppose, a genuine benefit to the celebrity life, is the unique social access it facilitates. In her book *Starstruck: The Business of Celebrity*, Elizabeth Currid-Halkett suggests that being a celebrity is like belonging to a members-only club. "They are a part of a very elite invite-only network," Currid-Halkett writes. Indeed, this celebrity club is a real and measurable phenomenon. Currid-Halkett's analysis of celebrity networks found that celebrities "exhibit just 3.26 degrees of separation from one another," far less than the well-known six degrees of separation. Celebrities hang together, know each other, and gravitate to the same social gatherings. Wanting entrance to this "club" and the perceived (and highly publicized) advantages it provides—private parties, movie premieres, award shows, and career-enhancing friendships—is an understandable goal.

But all this glamor and excitement will not, necessarily, make a person feel happier or more fulfilled. Nor will money. Research has consistently shown that after people hit middle-class levels of income, or slightly more, further increases in wealth do little to heighten happiness. Indeed, because of a process called hedonic adaptation, the thrill that these experiences and advantages provide quickly fades. As Fyodor Dostoyevsky astutely observed in the novel *The House of the Dead*: "Man is a pliable animal . . . a being who gets accustomed to everything." This includes, I am sure Fyodor would agree, getting a good table at a restaurant.

This phenomenon is supported by numerous empirical studies. One of the most famous, published in 1978, compared the happiness of twenty-two winners of major lotteries with that of twenty-nine paralyzed accident victims. Amazingly, the lottery winners were *not* happier and in fact took less pleasure in the ordinary aspects of life. While subsequent research has tweaked these results, the general premise—that people tend to revert to a kind of "happiness baseline" regardless of circumstances—has been experimentally replicated many times. This process may be an evolutionary adaptation that causes the stimuli we face day to day, whether it is an awesome Paleolithic cave, an attractive spouse, or a new Lamborghini, to fade into the background. This allows us to concentrate on novel stimuli, which are usually, from a survival point of view, the better use of our mental resources. Also, if we did not adapt to new circumstances, we would not continue to strive for new achievements, a compulsion that may also have evolutionary benefits. This adaptation happens regardless of the positive (marriage, a birth) or negative (a death in the family, divorce) nature of the event. Our subjective well-being requires us to adapt to whatever the circumstances are. While people often do not fully rebound from all negative events (unemployment, the onset of a disability), we are generally remarkably resilient. And people seem to adapt more consistently and completely to positive events. No matter how big the achievement, perk, or reward, the boost in happiness doesn't last long, and our level of happiness returns to the baseline. So, while getting a great table at a restaurant, traveling first class, hanging with other celebs, and going to movie premieres is exciting at first, the buzz diminishes. Then, remarkably quickly, the perks don't seem like perks, and they do little to boost happiness.

Ambition is another highly relevant reason people rapidly adapt to positive events. As soon as a goal is achieved—landing a new job, getting a part in a movie—people have a tendency to look for the next rung on the ladder leading to success and happiness. Research has found that having lofty aspirations is a predictor of *lower* well-being, especially if those aspirations relate to extrinsic goals (money, fame, rewards) and not intrinsic goals (self-acceptance, community feeling). Katherine Bao, who studies happiness at Manhattanville College, cautions that the relationship between aspirations and happiness is complex. For example, people with high aspirations are often happy, but, as Bao told me, "at some point aspirations may become so high that they are essentially impossible to achieve, and our research shows that when people fail to fulfill their aspirations, their happiness declines."

Another study, published in 2012, involved about five hundred students and revealed that constantly aspiring for *more* happiness equated with decreased happiness in the present. The authors, psychologists Kennon Sheldon and Sonja Lyubomirsky, concluded that "striving for ever-greater happiness may set one on a hedonic treadmill to no-where." Once again, the observation seems particularly relevant to our reach-for-the-stars society and for those seeking the essentially unattain-able goal of celebrity, which, for most, truly is a treadmill to nowhere.

THE DISADVANTAGES TO being a celebrity are generally well known. They are the stuff of headlines and celebrity biographies. They serve as fodder for entertainment journalists and gossip columnists. Much of Perez Hil-ton's online success, for instance, is built on mapping the misfortunes of celebrities. So it is worth considering why the negatives do not, in the eyes of aspiring celebrities, overwhelm the positives. Why don't people worry about all the bad stuff associated with fame? The biggest reason, I suspect, is one I have already described: optimistic bias. People simply do not think that bad things are going to happen to them. And they see their future in an overly optimistic light: they believe their chance of achieving a desired goal is better than average and are terrible at guessing what it will be like when they achieve it. "When *I* become a celebrity," the thinking goes, "I will get all the benefits and none of the bad stuff. I won't blow my money. I will appreciate my good fortune. I will be able to handle fame. I will stay in a good relationship. I will not have addiction problems." And on and on.

Daniel Gilbert, a professor of psychology at Harvard University, has spent decades studying and writing about why individuals make particular life choices and how those choices get screwed up. He has demonstrated that, sure enough, people overestimate their chance of success. In general, our view of what life will be like once our goals are achieved is overwhelm-ingly positive and largely inaccurate. "Few people see the negative conse-quences of being a celebrity. They fail to imagine all the complications of celebrity life," Gilbert tells me. "They don't think about the day-to-day reality—how they live their lives." In part, this is because we are constantly bombarded by unrealistic representations of celebrity existence. Pictures of celebrity homes, fashion, parties, and cars are absolutely everywhere. This plays into a number of our cognitive biases. For example, as Gilbert has noted in his research, if something is easy to imagine—say, a fabulous lifestyle—you may think it is more likely to happen than a more objective assessment would dictate. This tendency is tied to several cognitive biases, including confirmation bias and the availability heuristic (the ease to which we can bring something to mind), among others.

I decide to test my theory that a constant bombardment of positive representations of celebrity life feeds our cognitive biases. I walk into a bookstore and go to the entertainment section of the magazine stand. My goal is to pick up every magazine that covers celebrities and see if I can find in each at least one story that highlights the fabulous celebrity lifestyle, such as a feature about a spectacular house, vacation home, or apartment. To document my work, I intend to take a picture of both the cover of the magazine and the relevant story. I confess that the thoroughness of my investigation is seriously hampered by the embarrassing nature of my task.

"Excuse me, can I help you?" a young female clerk asks me as I start collecting my "data."

Picture how this must look to her. I am a middle-aged man awkwardly taking camera-phone pictures of starlets, some in bikinis, on the covers of gossip magazines. "I am, um, doing research . . . kind of," I reply. She clearly does not believe me but slowly walks away. She gives me one last over-the-shoulder glare. I forge ahead but get through only nine magazines before shame overwhelms me. Here are the results of my clumsy investigation:

HELLO! Magazine: "Kim Wilde [a UK pop star/presenter/model]: Inviting Us into Her Stunning 16th Century Retreat."

US Weekly: A bikini-clad Kim Kardashian is on the cover (I can't escape this woman). She is "slamming the fat bullies" for their mean comments about her pregnancy physique and with the headline declaring, "My Body Is Back, No Gimmicks, No Surgery." It is portrayed as a triumph. Revenge. A quick flip through the magazine reveals no stories that are explicitly about celebrity domiciles, but there is one on Jennifer Aniston's most recent holiday bash. That's close enough.

Life & Style Weekly: This has an article headlined the "Fabulous Life of Blake Lively." It includes a detailed description of her $2.35 million "Cosy Country Retreat," to which she is "putting personal touches" because "Martha Stewart is her idol."

People: As a regular reader, I have seen dozens of stories about celebrity homes. It is almost a regular feature. Indeed, by my rough calculations, more than 80 percent of its issues have at least one story about a cool celebrity home, vacation, and so on. In the issue I hold in the bookstore, the best example is a story entitled "The Jolie-Pitts: Australian Adventures" about how the "most glamorous party of eight" spends its time Down Under. (As I write this, People.com also has an online quiz entitled "Insane Celebrity Homes! From multimillion-dollar estates to homes with moats (seriously!)." It encourages us to take the test to find out "how well you know the domiciles of the rich and famous!" I clearly don't. Despite more than a year of immersion in celebrity culture, I get every question wrong.)

In Touch: This magazine, like so many others of this genre, takes a yin-yang approach to celebrity life. The cover has a headline that reads "I'm Lucky to Be Alive: Drugs, Arrests, Psych Wards . . ." The story is about the troubled life of former child star Amanda Bynes. But things get much more cheery later with a feature called "Crib of the Week." The story is about the actors Diane Kruger (*Troy, Inglourious Basterds*) and Joshua Jackson (*Fringe, Dawson's Creek*), who are selling their Hollywood "hillside hideaway," despite having fabulous neighbors such as Drew Barrymore, Zac Efron, and Katy Perry.

Star: This publication has a piece on Ricky Martin's $8.3 million high-rise pad in Manhattan, which, I am sure, affords Ricky many opportunities to live *la vida loca.*

Closer Weekly: I had never heard of this periodical. The catchphrase above the title says its goal is to bring me closer to the stars I love. As a result of this unabashed embrace of voyeurism, the magazine naturally has much on celebrity lifestyles, including a six-page spread on Jeff Probst's home or, as he calls it, "the house that *Survivor* built."

Scandalous: This big, glossy magazine looks like a one-off publication focused on the reckless lifestyles of the rich and famous (so, basically, a magazine about divorce, breakdowns, drugs, bankruptcy, and arrests). But I am including it on this list because it has an article entitled "Rehab Retreats for the Rich and Famous." One of these facilities, the magazine claims, costs $60,000 a month.

Of course, this is a survey of just one magazine stand and the stories that cover the amazing places where celebrities live. I could have undertaken a similar survey focused on clothes. There is almost always a best-dressed section in these magazines. Another big theme: celebrity kids. It seems as if every edition of *People* has a two-page photo spread showing celebrities hanging with their adorable children. Or I could have looked at TV shows or Twitter feeds from sources like TMZ or E! Online.

It is no surprise, Gilbert explains, that people would be enticed by these representations. "There is no reason to believe that social comparison theory doesn't apply to [individuals looking up to] celebrities," he observes. In other words, we upward compare to the fantasy world created by lifestyle reporting. Compared to the celebrity homes portrayed in entertainment magazines, most of us live in relative deprivation. And, as with beauty and body image, social media both intensify and increase the availability of images that play into our cognitive biases. Formats like Facebook and Twitter "bring us closer to celebrities," Gilbert says. Recent studies consistently show the power of new media to increase the sway of celebrity culture, for good and bad. "They are a stage for bragging. 'Look what I've got!'" Gilbert says. "This makes us feel bad. Most aspirations are set by looking around and seeing what others have."

And, if you believe what you see in social media and the entertainment media, celebrities have a lot!

THE QUEST FOR fame often starts in our teen years, and this ties into another reason why the downsides of celebrity life have little effect on our society's endemic quest for fame. Teenagers are notoriously oblivious to risk—particularly if the risk is likely to manifest in the far future. As biological entities, teenagers are pretty focused on the here and now. As the philosopher Adam Smith famously noted, "The contempt of risk and the presumptuous hope of success are in no period of life more active than at the age at which young people choose their professions."

A large body of research has backed up Smith's eighteenth-century observation. Some studies, for example, suggest that the teenage brain is wired to take on risks or, at least, perceives them differently than adult brains do. It is no surprise, then, that teenagers are willing to do some pretty crazy and dangerous things to achieve celebrity status. According to one study, for instance, 57 percent of adolescents already taking steroids would take a pill or supplement in order to achieve future sports success even if they were sure it would shorten their life. There is little evidence that the well-publicized risks associated with concussions in football and hockey have dissuaded any rising stars from playing. And UK teachers told researchers that becoming a celebrity is often a primary goal for their teenage students. Indeed, many of their students are willing to quit school to achieve it—which, I would suggest, is a fairly high-risk career strategy.

I can relate to this kind of risk taking. I was certain I was going to make it in the music industry. That certainty crystallized in my late teens. My mom—who provided advice in a very hands-off manner, parenting mostly by stealth—was supportive of my music aspirations but constantly pushed education. "Do whatever makes you happy," she would say, "but promise me you will get a university education." I came close to breaking that promise on several occasions. The pressure to hit the road with a struggling band emerged almost every year while I pursued my undergraduate degree. Sometimes I wonder what would have happened if I didn't hate being in a moving vehicle as much as I do. Did my fear of motion sickness keep me in school?

Back in West Hollywood, Arngrim muses on the attraction fame has for children and adolescents. "When you are a kid, it is normal to dream," Arngrim says. "But grownups are supposed to know it is nuts." The combination of adolescent risk taking and a deep parental belief that is skewed by various cognitive biases has likely propelled many an individual toward the search for celebrity status.

Paul Petersen could not agree more. "Why would parents wish this on their kids? Human beings have blinders on." Like Arngrim, Petersen knows Hollywood and what it is like to be famous. He started his acting career on *The Mickey Mouse Club* when he was just ten. He has been in a movie with Cary Grant and Sophia Loren and was on the popular *Donna Reed Show* from 1958 to 1966. More important for my purposes, he is the founder of an organization called A Minor Consideration, whose goal is to provide guidance and support for young performers. (Visitors to its website will find, among other sensible recommendations, that "child stars must pick their parents with care.") As the foundation's head, Petersen has had the opportunity to work closely with many young celebrities, past and present. He also aims to educate parents about the business ("it is show *business*, not show *fun*"); about the reality of making it (few can sustain a long career because, he says, "you *will* fall out of fashion"); and about all the lifestyle risks. He wants parents and children to know that "when you sacrifice the developmental years of your life, you will pay the price." But despite his best efforts, his message often does not get through. "Parents always think they can do it . . . beat the odds. Parents think the bad things won't happen. They ignore the advice."

Form Letter for Nutty Parents

Dear "Committed" Parent at My Kid's Hockey/Dance/Music/Whatever Class:
Re: The Nurturing of Your Kid's "Special" Talents

I realize that you want the best for your kid. I realize that you believe he/she is uniquely talented. My kids are super amazing too (except most of the time). But I am not sure you have thought through your plans for world domination in [hockey/ football/singing/dance/whatever]. Let's do the math. (1) The chance of making it big is approximately zero. Do not let confirmation bias fool you. Your kid is not going to be a world-renowned star. It is not going to happen. (2) Even if it does happen (and I can't emphasize this enough: it probably won't), there is a good chance that he/she will be divorced, broke, and unemployed before the age of thirty. [Note: If the kid is in hockey or football, add "head-injured," and if in popular music, add "struggling with addiction."] Also, perhaps most important, research tells us there is a good chance your child will not be happy. You are, in effect, wishing for your kid a life of financial misery, isolation, and lost opportunities. Is this a good idea?

I fully appreciate that I am coming off like a patronizing know-it-all jerk and that you will likely feel compelled to punch me in the face the next time you see me. Please don't. I have a delicate jaw. And besides, this letter was actually [neighbor's name] idea.

Yours truly,
[If brave, your name here. If not, insert spouse's name.]

PS: I understand from [neighbor's name] that you were a pretty good [hockey player/ football player/dancer/singer/whatever]. Sorry that didn't work out for you.

Individuals often strive for celebrity status because their parents have nudged them in that direction. And, no surprise, this often happens because parents want to live vicariously through their kids. A study published in 2013 provides the first empirical data on the idea that parents use their children to fulfill their own broken dreams. "Parents may come to see their children as symbols for their own success," the authors write, "and desire them to fulfill the ambitions they once held for themselves." It was a relatively small experiment, involving just seventy-three parents, for such a complex topic. Its authors focused on what the parents had to say about their ambitions for their children, rather than tracking actual parental behaviors. Nevertheless, the study provides empirical support for the notion that parents see their children as extensions of themselves and transfer to their children their own failed attempts at glory.

Most of us will recognize this phenomenon from our own experience. Many of us have seen it play out in hockey rinks, where we see little kids with $300 hockey sticks; at dance studios, where stage mothers primp two-year-olds; and at music recitals, where parents encourage their prodigies to spend more time practicing than sleeping. Other studies have found that people regret lost opportunities more than anything else. Nothing burns like the memory of an unfulfilled dream. So the compulsion to make up for lost opportunities through our children is hardly surprising.

And that reminds me: Why the heck won't any of my kids start a rock band? They'd be great!

THREE HOURS AFTER we started our discussion, Arngrim is still laughing, smiling, and willing to chat. The woman has a million stories. All good. I am sure Nellie would not have been so generous with her time or half as fun to hang out with. Arngrim tells me she is now happy. Her life is a satisfying mix of performing, writing, standup comedy (a routine built around her persona as a "prairie bitch"), and work as an AIDS activist. She has learned to embrace her Nellie past. She can't run from it, as I saw during our afternoon together, so she has found a constructive place for Nellie to hang. Perhaps not right on her shoulder but never far from view.

Before we part, I want to ask her one last question. As I have discussed, the combination of social pressure to "reach for the stars" and a host of built-in cognitive biases creates an environment that has made celebrity seem both worthwhile and attainable. But everything is an illusion, from the chance of making it to what it will be like if it is achieved. In other words, much of our culture, many of our dreams, and many of our life decisions flow from a foundation of promises and presumptions that are, in fact, no more real than the magic of the Wizard of Oz. Given this reality, I ask Arngrim, why do people try?

"You know, it is just ridiculous. It [success] is just so very rare," Arngrim says emphatically.

"But people like to gamble, even if they don't think of it that way?"

"Hey, I still buy lottery tickets, but I don't spend the rent," Arngrim says. "If people gambled with this kind of money in Vegas, everyone would say they had a gambling problem. But, for some reason, when people do it for fame and celebrity, for some bizarre reason, our society says it is OK."

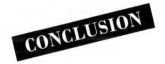

The Dream Crusher?

I have explored the myriad ways celebrity culture presents an inaccurate or warped picture of the world. I have tried to show the degree to which celebrities—or, really, the messages that flow from celebrity culture—are wrong about almost everything, whether in relation to health, beauty, the goals to which we should aspire, or definitions of the good life. But I have said little about the place, role, and impact of celebrity culture in society more broadly—and there is much that can be said (and many terrific scholars have had their say) on this point. Celebrity culture is, of course, more than just an interest in celebrities. It is a reflection of our collective values and a manifestation of complex interplay between social expectations and socioeconomic realities. As sociologist Karen Sternheimer writes in *Celebrity Culture and the American Dream*, "Rather than simple superficial distractions, celebrity and fame are unique manifestations of our sense of American social mobility: they provide the illusion that material wealth is possible for anyone. . . . Celebrities seem to provide proof that the American Dream of going from rags to riches is real and attainable."

This is more than mere academic musing. A belief in the celebrity illusion can have a tangible impact on life choices. A 2002 study of US college football players, to cite one more example, found that 84 percent

of the African American players had an "expectation of a career in professional athletics" and that 40 percent believed sports is the best route
to economic success. Keep in mind that these are individuals who were
in a university. One would hope they'd have a positive view of the role
of education in their future. The researchers also found that those players who held these kinds of beliefs were also more likely to have "been
placed on academic probation and suspension," among other less-than-
ideal behaviors.

Given what I've covered in this book, findings of this nature are far
from surprising, but they remain no less disheartening. Belief in celebrity
success is built on a foundation of lies, illusions, and empty exhortations
of the reach-for-the-stars variety. The chance of making it celebrity big
in any kind of celebrity-oriented career hovers near zero. And even if an
individual makes it big, the attainment of the goal is unlikely to provide
the promised long-term wealth or, more important, the desired happiness and well-being. There is no pot of gold at the end of the rainbow.

The misconceptions that exist in the context of health and beauty are
just as insidious. The beauty standard set by celebrity culture is not only
unrealistic; it also is increasingly disconnected from reality. This standard
has less and less to do with what humans actually look like. The bulk of
health and beauty products and recommendations peddled by or through
celebrities are either useless or harmful or both. They may also divert
millions of individuals from engaging in the simple and evidence-based
steps necessary to live in a health-promoting manner. Celebrity culture
places aesthetics above health and well-being; immediate results above
the adoption of sustainable, long-term health strategies; and, perhaps
worst of all, confuses science and pseudoscience, making it more difficult
for us all to sift through the mountains of health, diet, and beauty advice
that permeates popular culture.

The good news is that we can do things to improve our health and
even our appearance. We can adopt a healthy lifestyle that embraces
well-known and evidence-based practices that will have a measurable impact. And we can simply disregard the pseudoscientific spin that spews

from the celebrity universe. With few exceptions, it is all bunk. Ignore the diets. Ignore the fitness routines. Ignore the health and beauty advice.

But we should also consider strategies to mitigate the adverse impact that celebrity culture might have on our ambitions, our definition of success, and the way we view our current life circumstances. Simply by learning to recognize, and remind ourselves of, the numerous cognitive biases that twist how we think about the world may help us to make more informed life choices.

It is worth remembering, even if we don't really crave celebrity status, that celebrity culture can still have a significant impact on our life, by, for example, reinforcing a particular definition of success—the obtainment of wealth, a particular norm of beauty, and the like—that may tend to make us dissatisfied with our lot and to crave things that have little connection to happiness or health. Social comparisons, even to celebrity life, likely happen automatically. I am not arguing that we should settle for mediocrity, but perhaps we should occasionally critically appraise the nature of the goals for which we strive. Do they, for example, even exist?

"Jeez, Dad. You are kind of a downer," my oldest son, Adam, told me when we were talking about some of the themes in this book. "I am going to call you the dream crusher!"

With all due respect to my son, I think he is entirely wrong. I am not denying that it is fun to dream. Nor am I suggesting that if you really want to be a singer, actor, model, dancer, or professional athlete, you shouldn't aspire to that goal. But know the reality of the situation. And pursue the goal because you love the activity, the craft, or the challenge, not because you want to be rich and famous. This is advice I heard again and again while working on this book. I heard it from an *American Idol* finalist, a TV producer, directors, a legendary publicist, academics, award-winning actors, and many, many musicians. I view this advice not as dream crushing but as liberating. You aren't going to be rich and famous. Stop worrying about it.

Filmmaker and comedian Bobcat Goldthwait, whose 2011 film, *God Bless America*, includes a spoof of *American Idol*, provided this advice during a commencement speech he delivered for the college graduation of his daughter's class. "I truly believe that success is for creeps. We already reward narcissism way too much in our culture," he said. "Do what makes you happy, and be nice."

I'D LIKE TO END by reflecting on how all this fits into a bigger picture. I admit up front that only a thin strand of current data can be found to support the speculation that follows. But bear with me. I think this analysis provides an interesting context for thinking about the role and impact of celebrity culture in modern society.

The countries that seem the most obsessed with celebrity culture (i.e., the United States, United Kingdom, South Korea) do not score particularly high in rankings of population happiness. According to the 2013 *World Happiness Report*, a study prepared for the United Nations, the happiest countries in the world are Denmark, Norway, and Switzerland. Canada ranks sixth. The United States and the United Kingdom, two countries that both produce and consume a great deal of celebrity culture, rank seventeenth and twenty-second, respectively. These same celebrity-loving countries also have a terrible record when it comes to social mobility. The United Kingdom ranks last among the thirty-four nations in the Convention on the Organisation for Economic Co-operation and Development (OECD), and the United States is third from last. In other words, in these countries, moving up the socioeconomic ladder is nearly impossible. If you are born into poverty, you are likely to stay in poverty. If you are a middle-class kid, chances are you will be a middle-class adult. Ditto your kids. (Incidentally, the country that has the highest degree of social mobility? Happy Denmark.)

Some commentators have gone so far as to call the American dream a myth, a topic I discussed with Howard Steven Friedman, a well-known statistician with the United Nations and author of *The Measure of a Nation*. "The idea of social mobility, of becoming rich, is core to the American mythology," Friedman says. "But, ironically, American performance in this area is consistently one of the worst of the developed nations."

Friedman has observed that the statistics are depressing for those "who subscribe to the notion that America is a meritocracy and a 'land of opportunity.'" And the data tell us social mobility is getting worse.

What is the best way to ensure improved social mobility, a societal goal we can all agree is important? Education. A 2012 study by the PEW Charitable Trust, *Pursuing the American Dream: Economic Mobility Across Generations*, found that "a four-year college degree promotes upward mobility from the bottom and prevents downward mobility from the middle and top." I ask Erin Currier, the project director for PEW's Economic Mobility Project and a coauthor of the study, if education is the most important tool in the promotion of social mobility. "Absolutely. Research has shown this again and again," she says. "And what is often overlooked is that it leads not only to more mobility but better jobs." Given this reality, it is worth noting that numerous studies, such as the OECD's regular Programme for International Student Assessment, have consistently found that the US and UK education systems do not rank particularly well in comparison to those of other developed nations.

What do all these data about happiness, education, and social mobility have to do with celebrity culture? We live in a world where people increasingly turn to celebrity culture as a way of thinking about and striving for social mobility, whether through real life choices or merely through fantasies about a life that could be, and as a means of improving our well-being, health, and appearance. Is it a coincidence that countries that fare relatively poorly with respect to social mobility, happiness, and education also embrace celebrity culture and a reach-for-the-stars mentality? Perhaps. (I realize I am straying precariously close to an "opiate of the masses" thesis.) It seems hard to deny that a convergence of a variety of socioeconomic (e.g., poor social mobility) and technological (e.g., social media) trends with human psychological and social predispositions and biases has created the perfect conditions for celebrity culture to thrive.

I run this theory by Stephen Duncombe, a professor of media studies at New York University and author of *Dream: Re-Imagining Progressive Politics in an Age of Fantasy*. "This certainly seems plausible," he says.

"Celebrity is so tied to democracy and succeeding, especially now. People like Kim Kardashian seem real. They act like us. They come from places that we come from. This isn't Grace Kelly. Celebrity culture makes social mobility look like magic." Indeed, it is often sold as magic. It is sold as a life-changing process that is now—or so the celebrity myth goes—increasingly available to all.

Joshua Gamson, a professor at the University of San Francisco's College of Arts and a well-known commentator on celebrity culture, tells me something similar. "In a society with tremendous income inequality, with many avenues [to success] effectively closed, here you have a way to fantasy—a get-rich-quick fantasy. You can understand why people want to keep the dream alive," he says. "The shortcut to mobility is very appealing."

Currier agrees with the take presented by Gamson and Duncombe: "It is possible that, given the barriers to social mobility, for some, they see celebrity as the only viable option." To support this view, Currier tells me of a 2006 study that found 38 percent of those with annual incomes of less than $25,000 think that winning the lottery represents the most practical way for them to accumulate wealth. Given this kind of thinking, which, as Currier noted, is likely a manifestation of a perceived lack of options, is it any surprise that so many perceive that making it celebrity big is a viable goal? We could certainly quibble about the degree to which the rise in celebrity culture is a contributing cause or a by-product of existing social realities. But no matter how tenuous the connection or complex the direction of the relationship, it seems difficult to deny that our current fascination with celebrity has the potential to lead to more unhappiness—about our bodies, faces, clothes, careers, homes, virtually everything. More important, this societal obsession does little to elevate or prioritize activities that will promote true social mobility and well-being. The power of celebrity culture to distract in a less-than-constructive manner happens at the level of both the individual (e.g., decisions about education paths, the way we think about and define success, the use of individual and family resources, and so on) and society (e.g., how the public engages with broader social issues).

A study published in 2007 found that those who "follow celebrity culture are the least engaged in politics and least likely to use their social networks to involve themselves in action or discussion about public-type issues." There is, of course, a causation issue with this kind of data. (Perhaps those who aren't interested in social issues are attracted to celebrity culture?) Still, it shows that, at a minimum, celebrity culture does little to help or, as the authors note, the data challenges "suggestions of how popular culture might contribute to effective democracy."

On a more fundamental level, research suggests that celebrity culture has contributed to the rise of a more narcissistic society. Few have done as much work on this point as Jean Twenge, a psychologist at San Diego State University and coauthor of the 2009 book *The Narcissism Epidemic*. In a 2013 paper, she writes, "The overwhelming majority of the evidence shows that more recent generations of young people have more positive self-views, endorse more narcissistic personality traits, and are more self-focused." This attitude is the result of a number of factors, including our society's embrace of the reach-for-the-stars mentality and, as Twenge told me during a discussion about her work, "a celebrity world that showcases narcissism." Indeed, Twenge thinks popular culture has crossed the line and that such narcissistic traits now are viewed and portrayed as a good thing.

To be fair, not everyone agrees about the degree to which narcissism is actually increasing. But, regardless of the magnitude of the phenomenon—and I believe that the data, while still evolving, are pretty darn convincing—the implications could be significant. There is, for example, evidence that the current cohort of youth is more entitled and less interested in community and social engagements. (Note: This is not to say *every* youth has this disposition. I know many highly engaged and socially conscientious young people!) More than previous generations, they crave extrinsic rewards, such as fame, wealth, looks, and material possessions, and they are less interested in intrinsic rewards. Yet many studies tell us that a focus on intrinsic goals (such as community, personal growth, and relationships) is positively associated with indicators of psychological well-being and that an orientation toward extrinsic life goals is associated with decreased sense of well-being.

All that said, we need to take care not to place too much blame on the attractive shoulders of celebrities. We have bigger problems to solve, such as the growing economic disparity found throughout the world. Celebrity culture is a systemic phenomenon. Gwyneth may be a kook, but she didn't create the social and psychological conditions that give celebrity culture its considerable influence. As Sternheimer notes, celebrity culture is a "collective fantasy." It isn't imposed from above by Gwyneth, Pamela, *People*, or the Hollywood A-list. It is a force that both mirrors and shapes our hopes and desires, creating the compelling illusion that a transcendent beauty can be acquired and an elevating fame and fortune achieved by all. It seems that we are caught in a big, self-perpetuating celebrity-fueled cycle that goes something like this: Declining social mobility and diminishing life options lead to increasing dreams of celebrity fame and fortune. This, in turn, enhances the power and allure of celebrity, which causes a focus (perhaps with an ever-increasing narcissistic resolve) on extrinsic aspirations that lead to less happiness and distract us (and society more generally) from actions that may enhance social mobility, such as education and advocacy for social change.

It is, I admit, a rather grand claim. But it is not without foundation. As I have tried to show, we humans, whether we like it or not, are unusually interested in, and influenced by, celebrities and celebrity culture. And both the interest and their influence seem to be intensifying. At a minimum, we need to take steps to gain a greater appreciation of the long-term implications of this trend. And, perhaps most important, we need to strive collectively to put celebrity culture in its proper and entirely worthy place: as a fun and entertaining diversion.

Now would someone please hand me the latest issue of *People*?

I STARTED THIS JOURNEY through celebrity culture at an *American Idol* audition. I was surrounded by thousands of struggling singers who had the attainment of celebrity status as their primary motive. I had the opportunity to chat with dozens of these individuals. Many were making significant sacrifices in order to keep their dream alive. They told me, straight out, that fame was the goal. Did any succeed? Did any get even a moment of national TV exposure? Nope. But guess who did?

The week I am working on this concluding chapter is the same week, appropriately enough, that the new season of *American Idol* airs. I am excited to see whether any of the people I met at the audition made it in front of the judges. I am curious, for example, to see if Shakespeare Sunday will get to perform one of her original songs. Will the woman with pink hair finally get past the first round? Will the hoodie-wearing teenager start her climb out of poverty and toward fame and fortune? It is close to midnight when I finally find time to watch the episode I recorded earlier in the evening. It is a two-hour show and I am dead tired, so I fast-forward through much of the program, scanning the screen for a familiar face. I see nobody I know. No Shakespeare. No pink hair. No hoodie. But then, near the end of the show, I see a familiar face sticking out of a crowd. My face! I am on TV for half a second, perhaps less.

I freeze the image. Unlike the jubilant expressions on the young contestants that surround me in the shot, mine is an oddly pained look, as if I were drowning and gulping for air. The shock of seeing myself on TV causes me to call out. "I made it on *Idol!* Hey everyone, I'm on *American Idol!*"

"Shhhhh!" Joanne responds from upstairs. "Don't wake up the house."

"But, but . . . *I'm on American Idol*," I say to myself, lamely pointing at the TV screen and my frozen, contorted face.

ACKNOWLEDGMENTS

Because I was attempting to cover a lot of topics from a wide range of perspectives, I sought input from an eclectic range of academic experts. But I also wanted to move beyond the scientific literature in order to incorporate the views of individuals in the entertainment industry. As such, my first big thank-you goes to the many musicians, actors, writers, directors, and others—some successful, some struggling—who generously gave me their time and insights. Their participation was invaluable. Many of these individuals requested anonymity, often because they felt it would allow them to be more frank. The trade-off was worth it, I think. While many did not make it into the pages of this book, their candid stories informed much of my work and analysis.

Special thanks must also go to my good friend Tim Okamura. A renowned painter and a bit of celebrity in his own right, he connected me to many knowledgeable individuals, acted as an e-mail conduit for some of the interviews (e.g., Olivia Munn and Bryan Greenberg), and served as a sounding board for my many crazy ideas. Whether my query was about trying out for *Idol* or hanging with porn stars, his advice was always the same: go for it! I would similarly like to thank my brothers, Case and Sean, two of the brightest individuals around. Their constant support, suggestions, and encouragement are always hugely appreciated.

While researching this book I had the privilege to interview, correspond with, and/or interact with a wonderful assortment of individuals, including a member of the House of Lords (and I interviewed him *in* the House of Lords), world-famous actors, struggling but brilliant musicians, a Hollywood dermatologist, a celebrity physician, *American Idol* contestants, women who work in the adult entertainment business, and many others. It has been a unique and enormously entertaining ride. And I am incredibly grateful for their help. Without their involvement this book would not have been possible. So a massive thank-you to Annalise Acorn (University of Alberta), Lisa Leuschner Andersen (San Francisco), Pamela Anderson (Vancouver), Alison Arngrim (Los Angeles), Moses Avalon (Los Angeles), Katherine Bao (Manhattanville College), Kirk Barber (University of Calgary), Rhonda Bell (University of Alberta); Tanya Berry (University of Alberta), Marie Bertrand (Skin Science), Jessica Biesiekierski (KU Leuven), Arie Benchetrit (plastic surgeon, Montreal), Jennifer Blake (Society of Obstetricians and Gynaecologists of Canada), Susan Blond (New York), Norman Brown (University of Alberta), Joan Chrisler (Connecticut College), LuAnn Claps (New York), Erin Currier (Washington, DC), Chris de Gar (University of Alberta), Bob Demarco and Stephen Duncombe (New York University), Emme (New York), Nancy Etcoff (Harvard University), the Fabulous Calgary Sisters (a producer/writer and a lawyer in Hollywood), Chris Ferguson (Stetson University), Gary Fisher (University of Michigan), Yoni Freedhoff (Bariatric Medical Institute), Howard Steven Friedman (United Nations), Ramesh Ganeshram (New York), Curtis Gillespie (Edmonton), Joshua Gamson (University of San Francisco College of Arts), Peter Gibson (Monash University), Daniel Gilbert (Harvard University), Bryan Greenberg (New York), Christopher E. M. Griffiths (University of Manchester), Zach Hambrick (Michigan State University), Daniel S. Hamermesh (University of Texas), Steven Hoffman (McMaster University), Samuel J. Howard-Spink (New York University), A. J. Jacobs (New York), Camilla Knight (Swansea University), Lord Richard Layard (Centre for Economic Performance at the London School of Economics), Lainey Lui (gossip columnist and TV host), Karen Madsen (University of Alberta), Alice E. Marwick (Fordham University), Chris McCabe (University of Alberta), Linda McCarger (University of Alberta), Ben McConnell (former Beach House drummer—album: *Devotion*—Paris), Mary McDonough, Ashley Mears (Boston University), Tim Monich (everywhere, it seems), Amy Muise (University of Toronto), Olivia Munn (New York), Matthew Nisbet (American University), John O'Callaghan (Edmonton), Nan Okun (Maternal Fetal Medicine, University of Toronto), Dana Olstad (University of Alberta), Chris Peacocke (Edmonton), Tom Peacocke (Edmonton), T. W. Peacocke (Toronto), Ivona Percec (University of Pennsylvania), Paul Petersen (Hollywood), Rebecca Puhl (Yale University), Dhru Purohit (Los Angeles), Kim Raine (University of Alberta), Rhonda Rand (Hollywood), Donna Rockwell (New York), Jacques Romney (University of Alberta), David Sarwer (University of Pennsylvania), Jai Shah (McGill University), Tali Sharot (University College London), Emily Shores (McGill University), Michael Simkins (London), Jeremy Snyder (Simon Fraser University), Viren Swami (University of Westminster), James Turnbull (Korea), Leigh Turner (University of Minnesota), Jean Twenge (San Diego State University), Yalda T. Uhls (Children's Digital Media Center@LA), Vanessa and Elena ("the Valley"), Walter Willett (Harvard University), Kyla Wise (Vancouver), all the individuals who requested anonymity (specifically in New York and Hollywood), and anyone I forgot.

I also appreciate the continued support and help from my superb colleagues at the University of Alberta and the Health Law Institute, including Melissa Hartley, Ubaka Ogbogu, Maeghan Toews, Kalina Kaminova, Marianne Clarke, Amir Reshef, Erin Nelson, Nicki Baron, Christen Rachul, and, especially, Robyn Hyde-Lay, who delivered a continuous stream of useful research and ideas.

Thanks must also go to my wonderful agents, Chris Bucci and Anne McDermid. They provided much-needed encouragement and advice on scope and tone. I am also deeply indebted to Helene Atwan and everyone at Beacon Press for their support and their continued confidence in the relevance of my work. I would also like to acknowledge Helene for her terrific pull-no-punches editorial work. Not an easy task, I am certain.

I am thankful to the many funding agencies that have supported my research, including the Canada Research Chairs program, Trudeau Foundation, Alberta Heritage Foundation for Medical Research, Stem Cell Network (National Centres of Excellence), AllerGen (National Centres of Excellence), Genome Alberta, Canadian Institutes of Health Research, Social Sciences and Humanities Research Council, and the Alberta Policy Coalition for Cancer Prevention.

Finally, my biggest thanks must go to my long-suffering family. One theme of this book is that happiness and fulfillment do not come from wealth, material possessions, awards, career success, fame, or even recognition from your peers. It comes from the simple, day-to-day pleasures and, most important, from the people with whom you have the closest relationships. In this latter category, I have been truly blessed. So thank you, Adam, Alison, Jane, Michael, and Joanne. You are all superstars.

SELECTED REFERENCES
AND SOURCES

The references listed here are only a sample of the research, literature, and news items that I used while researching this book. For the sake of brevity, we felt a complete list was not necessary. I encourage interested readers to go to www.beacon.org/IsGwynethbiblio for a much more comprehensive reference list, including short notes about the relevance of various studies, reviews, and policy documents.

In the text, I tried to include enough information so that the relevant study could be identified in the alphabetical lists that follow or at www.beacon.org/IsGwynethbiblio. For many references, I have also added a short description of its relevance. A huge amount of literature is available, and my reference lists are far from complete. Nevertheless, I hope they give the reader a sense of the work that informed my research. As you will note, material came from a variety of sources, including the popular press and celebrity blogs. News stories give a sense of how reporters present the particular topic or may have been sources for quotes or other information.

I did not use the real names of some individuals I interviewed or observed. Some asked me to do this. For others—such as the children I witnessed at the fashion and talent events—it did not seem necessary or appropriate to identify them by name.

Finally, I'd like to comment on the challenge of researching celebrity statements, beliefs, and actions. Many of these come from celebrity-focused magazines or blogs, or from the general pop culture universe.

I recognize that these are not necessarily perfect representations of reality. Indeed, the information may have been, for example, altered by a publicist or may be the speculation of a celebrity blogger. But given that the point of the book is to explore the impact of celebrity culture, it is the public face of celebrity that is most relevant—no matter how bizarre (bird-poop facial?).

INTRODUCTION: IDOL DREAMS

John W. Ayers et al., "Do Celebrity Cancer Diagnoses Promote Primary Cancer Prevention?," *Preventive Medicine* 58 (2014): 81–84, doi:10.1016/j.ypmed.2013.11.007.

Melissa A. Click et al., "Making Monsters: Lady Gaga, Fan Identification, and Social Media," *Popular Music and Society* 36 (2013): 360–79.

Jake Halpern, *Fame Junkies: The Hidden Truths Behind America's Favorite Addiction* (Boston: Mariner Books, 2007).

Joseph Henrich and Francisco J. Gil-White, "The Evolution of Prestige: Freely Conferred Deference as a Mechanism for Enhancing the Benefits of Cultural Transmission," *Evolution and Human Behavior* 22 (2001): 165–96.

S. J. Hoffman and C. Tan, "Following Celebrities' Medical Advice: Meta-Narrative Analysis," *British Medical Journal* 347 (2013): f7151. A nice review of the evidence surrounding the influence celebrities have on fans' health decisions.

Kalina Kamenova et al., "Angelina Jolie's Faulty Gene: Newspaper Coverage of a Celebrity's Preventive Bilateral Mastectomy in Canada, the United States, and the United Kingdom," *Genetics in Medicine* 16, no. 7 (2013): 522–28.

Lynn E. McCutcheon et al., "Conceptualization and Measurement of Celebrity Worship," *British Journal of Psychology* 93 (2002): 67–87.

T. Niederkrotenthaler et al., "Changes in Suicide Rates Following Media Reports on Celebrity Suicide: A Meta-Analysis," *Journal of Epidemiology and Community Health* 66 (2012): 1037–42.

Alexandra Robbins, "Celebrity Trend Uses Nutrients Hospitals Desperately Need," *Washingtonian*, July 29, 2013.

Philip J. Smith et al., "Parental Delay or Refusal of Vaccine Doses, Childhood Vaccination Coverage at 24 Months of Age, and the Health Belief Model," *Public Health Report* 126, supplement 2 (2011): 135–46.

"Viewpoint: Did Our Brains Evolve to Foolishly Follow Celebrities?," *BBC News*, June 25, 2013, www.bbc.co.uk/news/magazine-23046602.

CHAPTER 1: DIETING, GWYNETH, AND MY CLEANSE

C. A. Bahlai et al., "Choosing Organic Pesticides over Synthetic Pesticides May Not Effectively Mitigate Environmental Risk in Soybeans," *PLoS ONE* 5 (2010): e11250. Shows organic pesticides are no better, from an environmental perspective, than synthetic.

J. R. Biesiekierski et al., "No Effects of Gluten in Patients with Self-Reported Non-Celiac Gluten Sensitivity After Dietary Reduction of Fermentable, Poorly

Absorbed, Short-Chain Carbohydrates," *Gastroenterology* 145 (2013): 320. This terrific study explores the existence of gluten sensitivity.

———, "Is Gluten a Cause of Gastrointestinal Symptoms in People Without Celiac Disease?," *Current Allergy and Asthma Reports* 13 (2013): 631–38.

Diane Bourn and John Prescott, "A Comparison of the Nutritional Value, Sensory Qualities, and Food Safety of Organically and Conventionally Produced Foods," *Critical Reviews in Food Science and Nutrition* 42 (2002): 1. This review found no health benefits to organic food.

Krista Casazza et al., "Myths, Presumptions, and Facts About Obesity," *New England Journal of Medicine* 368 (2013): 2236.

Emanuele Cereda et al., "Weight Cycling Is Associated with Body Weight Excess and Abdominal Fat Accumulation: A Cross-Sectional Study," *Clinical Nutrition* 30 (2011): 718. The impact of dieting on fat accumulation.

Katherine Chubinskaya et al., eds., "Myth vs. Fact: Adrenal Fatigue," Hormone Health Network, August 2010, www.hormone.org/hormones-and-health/myth-vs-fact/adrenal-fatigue. The website of the Endocrine Society identifies as medical doctors the four editors of this statement about the evidence surrounding adrenal fatigue.

Roger Clemens and Peter Pressman, "Detox Diets Provide Empty Promises," *Food Technology* 59 (2005): 18. Includes a quote about the absurdity of detox diets.

Alan D. Dangour et al., "Nutritional Quality of Organic Foods: A Systematic Review," *American Journal of Clinical Nutrition* 90 (2009): 680–85.

Marie Bernardine Danhof-Pont et al., "Biomarkers in Burnout: A Systematic Review," *Journal of Psychosomatic Research* 70 (2010): 505. The authors write: "No potential biomarkers for burnout were found, largely due to the incomparability of studies."

W. Dickey and N. Kearney, "Overweight in Celiac Disease: Prevalence, Clinical Characteristics, and Effect of a Gluten-Free Diet," *American Journal of Gastroenterology* 101, no. 10 (2006): 2356–59.

Daniel V. DiGiacomo et al., "Prevalence of Gluten-Free Diet Adherence Among Individuals Without Celiac Disease in the USA: Results from the Continuous National Health and Nutrition Examination Survey 2009–2010," *Scandinavian Journal of Gastroenterology*, August 48 (2013): 921–25.

Christopher Dye, "Health and Urban Living," *Science* 319 (2008): 766.

Mark S. Eberhardt and Elsie R. Pamuk, "The Importance of Place of Residence: Examining Health in Rural and Nonrural Areas," *American Journal of Public Health* 94 (2004): 1682.

L. Elli, "Where's the Evidence for Gluten Sensitivity?," *British Medical Journal* 345 (2012): e7360.

Kendall J. Eskine, "Wholesome Foods and Wholesome Morals? Organic Foods Reduce Prosocial Behavior and Harshen Moral Judgments," *Social Psychology and Personal Science* 4 (2012): 251. Suggests that buying organic actually makes people less "moral" and altruistic.

Guillaume Fond et al., "Fasting in Mood Disorders: Neurobiology and Effectiveness. A Review of the Literature," *Psychiatry Research* 209 (2013): 253–58. Outlines the psychological effects of fasting/starvation.

Food and Drug Administration, *Consumer Health Information: A Glimpse at "Gluten-Free" Food Labeling*, August 2011, www.fda.gov/downloads/ForConsumers/ConsumerUpdates/UCM266206.pdf.

Joel Forman et al., "Organic Foods: Health and Environmental Advantages and Disadvantages," *Pediatrics* 130 (2012): e1406.

A. D. Furlan et al., "Acupuncture and Dry-Needling for Low Back Pain," *Cochrane Database of Systematic Reviews* (2005): CD001351. See more at http://summaries.cochrane.org/CD001351/acupuncture-and-dry-needling-for-low-back-pain#sthash.lKyvvIWF.dpuf.

Glenn A. Gaesser and Siddhartha S. Angadi, "Gluten-Free Diet: Imprudent Dietary Advice for the General Population?," *Journal of the Academy of Nutrition and Dietetics* 112 (2012): 1330. This review references the 2006 study of 371 celiacs.

Brittany Galla, "Katy Perry Didn't Drink Alcohol for Three Months, Went on Cleanse to Prep for Vogue Cover," *Us*, July 27, 2013.

Ina Garth et al., "Effect of Two Different Weight Loss Rates on Body Composition and Strength and Power-Related Performance in Elite Athletes," *International Journal of Sport Nutrition and Exercise Metabolism* 21 (2011): 97. A Norwegian study on muscle mass post-fast and with slow weight loss.

C. Gilsenan et al., "Do Organic Cherry Vine Tomatoes Taste Better Than Conventional Cherry Vine Tomatoes? A Sensory and Instrumental Comparative Study from Ireland," *Journal of Culinary Science & Technology* 10 (2012): 154.

J. A. Houchins et al., "Effects of Fruit and Vegetable, Consumed in Solid vs. Beverage Forms," *International Journal of Obesity* 37 (2013): 1109.

Jung Sun Lee et al., "Weight Loss and Regain and Effects on Body Composition: The Health, Aging, and Body Composition Study," *Journals of Gerontology, Series A, Biological Sciences and Medical Sciences* 65 (2010): 78. This study found that yo-yo dieting "may contribute to a net loss of lean mass in older men but warrant[s] further studies."

Joanne Levasseur and Vera-Lynn Kubinec, "Pesticide Residue Found on Nearly Half of Organic Produce," CBC News, January 8, 2014, http://www.cbc.ca/news/canada/manitoba/pesticide-residue-found-on-nearly-half-of-organic-produce-1.2487712.

Traci Mann et al., "Medicare's Search for Effective Obesity Treatments: Diets Are Not the Answer," *American Psychologist* 62 (2007): 220. Highlights the ineffectiveness of virtually all diets.

Caitlin Mason et al., "History of Weight Cycling Does Not Impede Future Weight Loss or Metabolic Improvements in Postmenopausal Women," *Metabolism* 62 (2013): 127. Found that a history of yo-yo dieting did not impair metabolism for future weight loss.

Nathalie Michels et al., "Relation Between Salivary Cortisol as Stress Biomarker and Dietary Pattern in Children," *Psychoneuroendocrinology* 38 (2013): 1512.

Ranit Mishori et al., "The Dangers of Colon Cleansing," *Journal of Family Practice* 60 (2011): 454. Outlines the lack of evidence to support the use of colon cleanses and similar treatments.

Jaakko Mursu et al., "Dietary Supplements and Mortality Rate in Older Women," *Archives of Internal Medicine* 171, no. 18 (2011): 1625–33.

Lisa M. Nackers et al., "The Association Between Rate of Initial Weight Loss and Long-Term Success in Obesity Treatment: Does Slow and Steady Win the Race?," *International Journal of Behavioral Medicine* 17 (2010): 161.

———, "Effects of Prescribing 1,000 Versus 1,500 Kilocalories per Day in the Behavioral Treatment of Obesity: A Randomized Trial," *Obesity* 21 (2013): 248.

Marion Nestle and Malden C. Nesheim, "To Supplement or Not to Supplement: The U.S. Preventive Services Task Force Recommendations on Calcium and Vitamin D," *Annals of Internal Medicine* 158 (2013): 701.

S. G. Newmaster et al., "DNA Barcoding Detects Contamination and Substitution in North American Herbal Products," *BMC Medicine* 11 (2013): 222. Highlights the poor quality of most supplements.

Steven Novella, "No Health Benefits from Organic Food," *Science-Based Medicine* (September 5, 2012), http://www.sciencebasedmedicine.org/no-health-benefits -from-organic-food/.

———, "Non-Celiac Gluten Sensitivity," *Neurologica* (blog), May 15, 2014. In this skeptical look at NCGS, the author concludes: "NCGS is probably not a real entity."

Keith O'Brien, "Should We All Go Gluten-Free?," *New York Times*, November 25, 2011.

Ian R. Reid et al., "Effects of Vitamin D Supplements on Bone Mineral Density: A Systematic Review and Meta-Analysis," *Lancet* 383 (2013): 136–55. This study shows limited or no benefit to vitamin D in the context of bone health.

J. Rodin et al., "Weight Cycling and Fat Distribution," *International Journal of Obesity* 14 (1990): 303. This study found that yo-yo dieting did have an impact on fat distribution.

Amy Roeder, "Skip the Juice, Go for Whole Fruit: Eating Whole Fruits, Particularly Blueberries, Grapes, Apples, Linked to Lower Risk of Type 2 Diabetes," *Harvard Gazette*, August 29, 2013, http://news.harvard.edu/gazette/story/2013/08/reduce -type-2-diabetes-risk/.

A. Catherine Ross et al., eds., *Dietary Reference Intakes for Calcium and Vitamin D* (Washington, DC: National Academies Press, 2011).

Gopal K. Singh and Mohammad Siahpush, "Widening Rural–Urban Disparities in Life Expectancy, U.S., 1969–2009," *American Journal of Preventive Medicine* 46 (2014): e19–e29. The authors write: "Life expectancy was inversely related to levels of rurality."

G. K. Singh et al., "All-Cause and Cause-Specific Mortality Among US Youth: Socioeconomic and Rural–Urban Disparities and International Patterns," *Journal of Urban Health* 90 (2013): 388. Showed rural youth were at greater risk.

Crystal Smith-Spangler et al., "Are Organic Foods Safer or Healthier Than Conventional Alternatives? A Systematic Review," *Annals of Internal Medicine* 157 (2012): 348. This Stanford study found no nutritional difference between organic and conventionally grown foods.

Victoria L. Stevens et al., "Weight Cycling and Mortality in a Large Prospective US Study," *American Journal of Epidemiology* 175 (2012): 785. The authors write: "These results do not support an increased risk of mortality associated with weight cycling [yo-yo dieting]."

Stephanie Strom, "Has 'Organic' Been Oversized?," *New York Times*, July 7, 2012, www.nytimes.com/2012/07/08/business/organic-food-purists-worry-about-big -companies-influence.html. This story outlines the degree to which the organic food industry has been taken over by "Big Food" companies.

Bianchi Talavera and Martin Jose, "Sensory Analysis of Pac Choi and Tomato Grown Under Organic and Conventional Systems," PhD diss., Kansas State University, 2009. The authors write: "There do not appear to be major sensory differences between organic and conventional products specific to the crops and seasons studied."

Evropi Theodoratou et al., "Vitamin D and Multiple Health Outcomes: Umbrella Review of Systematic Reviews and Meta-Analyses of Observational Studies and Randomised Trials," *British Medical Journal* 348 (2014): g2035. The authors write: "Highly convincing evidence of a clear role of vitamin D does not exist for any outcome."

A. Janet Tomiyama et al., "Low Calorie Dieting Increases Cortisol," *Psychosomatic Medicine* 72 (2010): 357.

Georgios Tsivgoulis et al., "Adherence to a Mediterranean Diet and Risk of Incident Cognitive Impairment," *Neurology* 80 (2013): 1684.

Alice Tuff and Harriet Bell, "The Voice of Young Science Network Brings You . . . The Detox Dossier," *Voice of Young Science*, 2009, www.senseaboutscience .org/data/files/resources/48/Detox-Dossier-Embargoed-until-0001-5th-jan -2009.pdf.

UK Food Standards Agency, *Comparison of Putative Health Effects of Organically and Conventionally Produced Foodstuffs: A Systematic Review*, 2009, http://multimedia .food.gov.uk/multimedia/pdfs/organicreviewreport.pdf. Concludes that there is no health benefit from organic food.

Catherine Ulbricht et al., "Caffeine Clinical Bottom Line: An Evidence-Based Systematic Review by the Natural Standard Research Collaboration," *Alternative and Complementary Therapies* 18 (2012): 324. A nice review of research on the benefits of coffee, including noting the lack of evidence for the use of caffeine to treat wrinkles and cellulite.

Rohini Vanga and Daniel A. Leffler, "Gluten Sensitivity: Not Celiac and Not Certain," *Gastroenterology* 145 (2013): 276. This editorial questions the existence of nonceliac gluten sensitivity.

S. J. Wallner et al., "Body Fat Distribution of Overweight Females with a History of Weight Cycling," *International Journal of Obesity* 28 (2004): 1143–48. This study finds different fat distribution in women with a history of weight cycling.

Elaine Watson, "Gluten Free 'Most Popular Approach to Weight Loss' for 2013," Food Navigator-USA.com, December 20, 2012, http://www.foodnavigator-usa.com /Markets/Gluten-free-most-popular-approach-to-weight-loss-for-2013-but-it -doesn-t-work-say-dietitians.

CHAPTER 2: BEAUTY TIPS FROM BEAUTIFUL PEOPLE

"Antiaging Products and Services: The Global Market," BCC Research, August 2013.

Henri-Jean Aubin, "Weight Gain in Smokers After Quitting Cigarettes: Meta-analysis," *British Medical Journal* 345 (2012): e4439.

John Axelsson et al., "Beauty Sleep: Experimental Study on the Perceived Health and Attractiveness of Sleep-Deprived People," *British Medical Journal* 341 (2010): c6614.

Gregory Barsh and Laura D. Attardi, "A Healthy Tan?," *New England Journal of Medicine* 356 (2007): 2208.

Corey Hannah Basch et al., "Improving Understanding About Tanning Behaviors in College Students," *Journal of the American College of Health* 60 (2012): 250. On practices and attitudes.

Elaina Bergamin et al., "Trends in Tobacco and Alcohol Brand Placements in Popular U.S. Movies, 1996 Through 2009," *Journal of American Medical Association Pediatrics* 167 (2013): 634.

F. P. Cappuccio et al., "Sleep Duration and All-Cause Mortality: A Systematic Review and Meta-Analysis of Prospective Studies," *SLEEP* 33 (2010): 585.

CDC, "Insufficient Sleep Is a Public Health Epidemic," Centers for Disease Control and Prevention (2011), www.cdc.gov/features/dssleep/. A review of research on sleep behavior in the United States.

A. Charlesworth, "Smoking in the Movies Increases Adolescent Smoking: A Review," *Pediatrics* 116 (2005): 1516.

N. Chen, et al. "Acupuncture for Bell's Palsy," *Cochrane Database of Systematic Reviews* (2010): CD002914. An example of a review that outlines the poor evidence base for the efficacy of acupuncture.

Arnaud Chiolero et al., "Consequences of Smoking for Body Weight, Body Fat Distribution, and Insulin Resistance," *American Journal of Clinical Nutrition* 87 (2008): 801. A good review of the impact of smoking on body weight. It refers to a paper showing that, over time, smokers and nonsmokers gain about the same amount of weight.

David Colquhoun and Steven P. Novella, "Acupuncture Is Theatrical Placebo," *Anesthesia and Analgesia* 116 (2013): 1360–63.

Janet M. Distefan et al., "Do Favorite Movie Stars Influence Adolescent Smoking Initiation?," *American Journal of Public Health* 94 (2004): 1239–44. This is a skeptical analysis of acupuncture.

Helen Dixon et al., "Portrayal of Tanning, Clothing Fashion and Shade Use in Australian Women's Magazines, 1987–2005," *Health Education Research* 23 (2008): 791.

Kathryn Doyle, "Tobacco on TV Tied to Adult Smoking Rates," Reuters, April 15, 2014, www.reuters.com/article/2014/04/15/us-tv-tobacco-rates-idUSBREA3E1IA20140415.

Daisy Dumas, "So That's Her Secret! Gwyneth Paltrow Reveals Her Favourite Anti-Ageing Beauty Trick," *Daily Mail* (UK), July 29, 2011.

Anthony Elliott, "'I Want to Look Like That!': Cosmetic Surgery and Celebrity Culture," *Cultural Sociology* 5 (2011): 463.

John Ericson, "Time for Beauty Rest: Skin Aging Linked to Lack of Sleep," *Medical Daily*, July 23, 2013, www.medicaldaily.com/articles/17705/20130723/sleep-aging -skin-beauty-rest-estee-lauder.htm.

Gary J. Fisher et al., "Looking Older: Fibroblast Collapse and Therapeutic Implications," *Archives of Dermatology* 144 (2008): 666. This is a terrific review of the evidence on antiaging therapies.

Yolanda R. Helfrich et al., "Effect of Smoking on Aging of Photoprotected Skin," *Archives of Dermatology* 143 (2007): 397. Among other things, this study demonstrates that "the degree of photoprotected skin aging correlates well with age and packs of cigarettes smoked per day."

Dawn M. Holman and Meg Watson, "Correlates of Intentional Tanning Among Adolescents in the United States: A Systematic Review of the Literature," *Journal of Adolescent Health* 52 (2013): 552. This study finds that wanting to look like a celebrity is associated with tanning behavior.

Maria Celia B. Hughes et al., "Sunscreen and Prevention of Skin Aging: A Randomized Trial," *Annals of Internal Medicine* 158 (2013): 781. A study on the antiaging benefits of sunscreen.

Nina G. Jablonski, "From Bardot to Beckham: The Decline of Celebrity," *Skin Cancer Foundation* 28 (2010): 42–44, www.skincancer.org/prevention/tanning/from -bardot-to-beckham-the-decline-of-celebrity-tanning. Reviews the nature and impact of the celebrity-inspired rise of suntanning behaviors.

Misbah H. Khan et al., "Treatment of Cellulite," *American Academy of Dermatology* 62 (2010): 373.

Suna Koh et al., "Importance-Performance Analysis with Benefit Segmentation of Spa Goers," *International Journal of Contemporary Hospitality Management* 22 (2010): 718. On the size and nature of the spa market (e.g., annual revenue of approximately $10 billion).

Julie Latreille et al., "Dietary Monounsaturated Fatty Acids Intake and Risk of Skin Photoaging," *PLoS One* 7 (2012): e44490.

Sagit Maier-Schwartz, "Bringing Beverly Hills Cosmetic Surgery to the Middle East," *Atlantic*, May 29, 2013, www.theatlantic.com/health/archive/2013/05/bringing -beverly-hills-cosmetic-surgery-to-the-middle-east/276302/.

Evgenia Makrantonaki, "Genetics and Skin Aging," *Dermatoendocrinology* 4 (2012): 280. A nice review on the role of genes and ethnicity in the context of skin.

Andrew Marszal, "Mad Men Boost for Lucky Strike Cigarettes Angers Campaigners," *Telegraph* (UK), September 22, 2013, www.telegraph.co.uk/health/healthnews /10326252/Mad-Men-boost-for-Lucky-Strike-cigarettes-angers-campaigners.html.

Andrew E. Mayes et al., "Environmental and Lifestyle Factors Associated with Perceived Facial Age in Chinese Women," *PLoS One* 5 (2010): e15270.

Mayo Clinic Staff, "Cellulite," Diseases and Conditions, *Mayo Clinic*, February 22, 2014, http://www.mayoclinic.org/diseases-conditions/cellulite/basics/definition /con-20029901.

Juan Meng and Po-Lin Pan, "Investigating the Effects of Cosmeceutical Product Advertising in Beauty-Care Decision Making," *International Journal of Pharmaceutical and Healthcare Marketing* 6 (2012): 250. How women make decisions about antiaging products. The study also says the global cosmetics market was more than $27 billion in 2010.

Rebecca Muckelbauer et al., "Association Between Water Consumption and Body Weight Outcomes: A Systematic Review," *American Journal of Clinical Nutrition* 98 (2013): 282.

Amy Muise and Serge Desmarais, "Women's Perceptions and Use of 'Anti-Aging' Products," *Sex Roles* 63 (2010): 126.

Ushma S. Neill, "Skin Care in the Aging Female: Myths and Truths," *Journal of Clinical Investigation* 122 (2012): 473. A terrific review of evidence associated with antiaging treatments and noting, for example, that several experts think spa facials do more harm than good.

Katherine Nolan and Ellen Marmur, "Over-the-Counter Topical Skincare Products: A Review of the Literature," *Journal of Drugs in Dermatology* 11 (February 2012): 220–24.

Gwyneth Paltrow, "The Knowledge: Gwyneth Paltrow on How to Create a Lean Body Shape," Telegraph.co.uk, July 29, 2013, http://fashion.telegraph.co.uk/beauty /news-features/TMG10204044/The-Knowledge-Gwyneth-Paltrow-on-how-to -create-a-lean-body-shape.html.

Panel on Dietary Reference Intakes for Electrolytes and Water, Institute of Medicine, *Dietary Reference Intakes for Water, Potassium, Sodium, Chloride, and Sulfate* (Washington, DC: National Academies Press, 2005), http://books.nap.edu /openbook.php?record_id=10925. A report on the amount of water required to maximize health. See also the press release with a relevant quote: "Report Sets Dietary Intake Levels for Water, Salt, and Potassium to Maintain Health and Reduce Chronic Disease Risk," www8.nationalacademies.org/onpinews/newsitem .aspx?RecordID=10925.

S. R. Patel, "Reduced Sleep as an Obesity Risk Factor," *Obesity Review* 10 (2009): 61. Shows that "reduced sleep appears to represent a novel, independent risk factor for increased weight gain."

Kurtis B. Reed et al., "Increasing Incidence of Melanoma Among Young Adults," *Mayo Clinic Proceedings* 87 (2012): 328–34.

Gretchen Reynolds, "Younger Skin Through Exercise," *New York Times, Well* blog, April 16, 2014, http://well.blogs.nytimes.com/2014/04/16/younger-skin-through -exercise/?_php=true&_type=blogs&_r=0. Reports on McMaster University research on the impact of exercise on skin health.

H. W. Rogers et al., "Incidence Estimate of Nonmelanoma Skin Cancer in the United States, 2006," *Archives of Dermatology* 146 (2010): 283–87.

Les Rose, "Do Further Studies on Acupuncture for Pain Make Sense? An Informal Review," *Focus on Alternative and Complementary Therapies* 18 (2013): 85. Shows that the effect size—that is, the clinical effect of the measured intervention—for acupuncture studies is small.

Harvey Simons, "Skin Wrinkles and Blemishes," University of Maryland Medical Center, 2012, http://umm.edu/health/medical/reports/articles/skin-wrinkles-and -blemishes. Excellent summary of the causes, prevention, and treatment of wrinkles.

Smart Tan, "Gwyneth Paltrow: Get Some Sun!," Smart Tan.com, June 21, 2010.

Nicholas P. Stamford, "Stability, Transdermal Penetration, and Cutaneous Effects of Ascorbic Acid and Its Derivatives," *Journal of Cosmetic Dermatology* 11 (2012): 310.

Telegraph, "Unhealthy Lifestyles 'Age a Woman's Skin by 10 Years,'" June 4, 2013, www .telegraph.co.uk/health/healthnews/10097752/Unhealthy-lifestyles-age-a-womans -skin-by-10-years.html.

F. Turati et al., "Efficacy of Cosmetic Products in Cellulite Reduction: Systematic Review and Meta-Analysis," *Journal of the European Academy of Dermatology and Venereology* 28 (2013): 1.

Melanie Wakefield et al., "Role of the Media in Influencing Trajectories of Youth Smoking," *Addiction* 98 (2003): 79. An excellent review of the complex role of media in smoking behavior, noting, among other things, that "the media act as a source of observational learning by providing models which teenagers may seek to emulate."

Sarah Ward, "Spa Industry Worth $255 Billion," *European Spa*, 2008, www .raisondetrespas.com/wp-content/uploads/2012/02/Global-Spa -business-2008.pdf.

R. Wolf et al., "Nutrition and Water: Drinking Eight Glasses of Water a Day Ensures Proper Skin Hydration—Myth or Reality? *Clinical Dermatology* 28 (2010): 380.

World Health Organization, "The Known Health Effects of UV," n.d., www.who.int /uv/faq/uvhealtfac/en/index2.html. A nice summary of the impact of UV light, including an emphasis on the fact that "there is no such thing as a healthy tan!"

———, "Tobacco," May 2014, www.who.int/mediacentre/factsheets/fs339/en/. Statistics on health risks associated with smoking.

CHAPTER 3: PAMELA ANDERSON'S BREASTS

AFP Relaxnews, "Double-Jaw Surgery Is the Latest Extreme Addition to South Korea's Plastic Surgery Fad," *New York Daily News*, May 28, 2013, www.nydailynews .com/life-style/health/s-korea-painful-beauty-fad-bone-cutting-jaw-surgery -article-1.1356287.

American Academy of Facial Plastic and Reconstructive Surgery, "Annual AAFPRS Survey Finds 'Selfie' Trend Increases Demand for Facial Plastic Surgery Influence on Elective Surgery," press release, March 2013, www.aafprs.org/media/stats_polls /m_stats.html.

American Society for Aesthetic Plastic Surgery, "Rising Demand for Female Cosmetic Genital Surgery Begets New Beautification Techniques," *PRWeb*, April 15, 2013, www.prweb.com/releases/plastic-surgery/04/prweb10614540.htm. Includes statistics on the number of cosmetic vagina surgeries.

Susan Carpenter, "Plastic Surgery—It's a Guy Thing Too," *Los Angeles Times*, April 15, 2012, http://articles.latimes.com/2012/apr/15/image/la-ig-male-plastic-surgery -20120415.

Nitin Chauhan et al., "Perceived Age Change After Aesthetic Facial Surgical Procedures," *Archives of Facial Plastic Surgery* 14 (2012): 258.

Curtis A. Fogel and Andrea Quinlan, "Lady Gaga and Feminism: A Critical Debate," *Cross-Cultural Communication* 7 (2011): 184–88. Questions the degree to which performers like Lady Gaga forward a feminist agenda, "generating unrealistic expectations of female empowerment."

James Griffith et al., "Pornography Actresses: An Assessment of the Damaged Goods Hypothesis," *Journal of Sex Research* 50 (2013): 621–32. One of the few studies to explore the attitudes of porn stars, including why they are attracted to the industry.

Daniel Hamermesh and Jeff Biddle, "Looks and the Labour Market," *American Economic Review* 84 (1994): 1174. One of Hamermesh's well-known studies on income and looks.

Daniel S. Hamermesh and Jason Abrevaya, "Beauty Is the Promise of Happiness," *European Economic Review* 64 (2013): 351. An international study on the direct and indirect impact of beauty on happiness.

Daniel S. Hamermesh et al., "Dress for Success: Does Primping Pay?," *Labour Economics* 9 (2002): 361.

Seunghwa Madeleine Han, "Pretty in Plastic: K-Pop and Korea's Plastic Surgery Boom," *New America Media*, December 30, 2012, http://newamericamedia.org /2012/12/pretty-in-plastic----k-pop-and-koreas-plastic-surgery-boom.php. This includes the quote on the percentage of teenagers getting plastic surgery and the desire to look like a K-pop star.

Harris Poll, "One in Five U.S. Adults Now Has a Tattoo," *Harris Interactive*, February 23, 2012, www.harrisinteractive.com/NewsRoom/HarrisPolls/tabid/447/mid/1508 /articleId/970/ctl/ReadCustom%20Default/Default.aspx.

Sotonye Imadojemu et al., "Influence of Surgical and Minimally Invasive Facial Cosmetic Procedures on Psychosocial Outcomes: A Systematic Review," *Journal of the American Medical Association Dermatology* 149 (2013): 1325–33.

International Society of Aesthetic Surgery, "Celebrity Influences on Plastic Surgery," 2008, www.isaps.org/. This survey ranked Pamela Anderson as the person with the most sought-after breasts by those seeking cosmetic surgery.

Barry Jones and Steven J. Lo, "How Long Does a Face Lift Last? Objective and Subjective Measurements over a 5-Year Period," *Plastic and Reconstructive Surgery* 130 (2012): 1317.

Kian Karimi et al., "The Efficacy of Rhinoplasty Alone in Facial Rejuvenation," *American Journal of Otolaryngology* 32 (2011): 269. The finding was that nose jobs alone were not rejuvenating.

B. Kelly and C. Foster, "Should Female Genital Cosmetic Surgery and Genital Piercing Be Regarded Ethically and Legally as Female Genital Mutilation?," *BJOG: An International Journal of Obstetrics & Gynaecology* 119 (2012): 389. Argues that genital cosmetic surgery should not be legal.

Mary Kosut, "An Ironic Fad: The Commodification and Consumption of Tattoos," *Journal of Popular Culture* 39 (2006): 1035.

Soohyung Lee and Keunkwan Ryu, "Plastic Surgery: Investment in Human Capital or Consumption?," *Journal of Human Capital* 6 (2012): 224. Concludes that cosmetic surgery does not improve looks sufficiently to make it worthwhile from an economic perspective.

Lih-Mei Liao and Sarah M. Creighton, "Female Genital Cosmetic Surgery: A New Dilemma for GPs," *British Journal of General Practice* 61 (2011): 7. Notes the risks and ethical issues associated with "designer vaginas."

Lih-Mei Liao et al., "An Analysis of the Content and Clinical Implications of Online Advertisements for Female Genital Cosmetic Surgery," *BMJ Open* 2 (2012).

J. Maltby and L. Day, "Celebrity Worship and Incidence of Elective Cosmetic Surgery: Evidence of a Link Among Young Adults," *Journal of Adolescent Health* 49 (2011): 483.

J. Margraf et al., "Well-Being from the Knife? Psychological Effects of Aesthetic Surgery," *Clinical Psychological Science* 1 (2013): 239. This study found most people were happy with the results of cosmetic surgery.

Lina Michala et al., "Female Genital Cosmetic Surgery: How Can Clinicians Act in Women's Best Interests?," *Obstetrician & Gynaecologist* 14 (2012): 203. The authors write: "There is limited evidence to allow women to give informed consent."

Alex Molotkow, "July Cover Star Olivia Munn on Geeks, Hollywood Jerks and Finding Love," *Flare*, June 7, 2013.

C. Moran and C. Lee, "What's Normal? Influencing Women's Perceptions of Normal Genitalia: An Experiment Involving Exposure to Modified and Nonmodified Images," *BJOG: An International Journal of Obstetrics & Gynaecology* 121, no. 6 (2013): 761–66.

Jacob E. Osterhout, "Seeking a Royal Sniffer: New York Women Rushing to Get the Kate Middleton Nose," *New York Daily News*, March 13, 2013, www.nydailynews .com/life-style/ny-women-rushing-kate-middleton-nose-article-1.1287848 #ixzz2cLexhR6L.

Jordi Quoidbach et al., "The End of History Illusion," *Science* 339 (2013): 96. This study explores how poor we are at predicting how much we change over time.

David B. Sarwer et al., "An Investigation of Changes in Body Image Following Cosmetic Surgery," *Plastic and Reconstructive Surgery* 109 (2002): 363. A study on the impact of plastic surgery on overall body image and happiness.

———, "Two-Year Results of a Prospective, Multi-Site Investigation of Patient Satisfaction and Psychosocial Status Following Cosmetic Surgery," *Aesthetic Surgery Journal* 28 (2008): 245.

Abhishek Seth, "How *Baywatch* Unknowingly Changed the World," *Huffington Post*, September 25, 2013, http://www.huffingtonpost.com/abhishek-seth/how-baywatch -unknowingly-changed-the-world_b_3891368.html.

Julie Slevec and Marika Tiggemann, "Attitudes Toward Cosmetic Surgery in Middle -Aged Women: Body Image, Aging Anxiety, and the Media," *Psychology of Women Quarterly* 34 (2010): Q65. The authors write that the "effects of media on cosmetic surgery attitudes were primarily direct."

Steffanie Sperry et al., "Cosmetic Surgery Reality TV Viewership," *Annals of Plastic Surgery* 62, no. 7 (2009). This study looked at the impact of shows like *Extreme Makeover*.

Surgical Practice Working Party, *Professional Standards for Cosmetic Practice* (London: Royal College of Surgeons of England, 2013), www.rcseng.ac.uk/publications /docs/professional-standards-for-cosmetic-practice/.

Viren Swami et al., "Acceptance of Cosmetic Surgery and Celebrity Worship: Evidence of Associations Among Female Undergraduates," *Personality and Individual Differences* 47 (2009): 869.

Stacey Tantleff-Dunn, "Breast and Chest Size: Ideals and Stereotypes Through the 1990s," *Sex Roles* 45 (2001): 231. Notes the role of Pamela Anderson.

A. Joshua Zimm et al., "Objective Assessment of Perceived Age Reversal and Improvement in Attractiveness After Aging Face Surgery," *JAMA Facial Plastic Surgery* 15 (2013): 405. This study found little improvement in appearance of age as a result of cosmetic surgery.

CHAPTER 4: WIRED BEHAVIOR

Michèle Belot et al., "Beauty and the Sources of Discrimination," *Journal of Human Resources* 47 (Summer 2012): 851. This is the TV-game-show study.

Katrina Bishop, "Abercrombie Hiring of Hot Staff Challenged in Europe," *CNBC*, July 29, 2013, www.cnbc.com/id/100921082.

Jeff Borland and Andrew Leigh, "Unpacking the Beauty Premium: What Channels Does It Operate Through, and Has It Changed Over Time?," *Economic Record* 90 (2012): 17–32.

Kyle Buchanan, "Leading Men Age, but Their Love Interests Don't," *Vulture*, April 18, 2013, www.vulture.com/2013/04/leading-men-age-but-their-love-interests-dont.html. This provides a terrific breakdown on the age gap between famous male-and-female onscreen couples.

Vanessa M. Buote et al., "Setting the Bar: Divergent Sociocultural Norms for Women's and Men's Ideal Appearance in Real-World Contexts," *Body Image* 8 (2011): 322.

M. Castillo, "The Benefits of Beauty," *American Journal of Neuroradiology* 34 (2013): 1.

Jill A. Cattarin et al., "Body Image, Mood, and Televised Images of Attractiveness: The Role of Social Comparison," *Journal of Social and Clinical Psychology* 19 (2000): 220.

Nancy Etcoff, *Survival of the Prettiest: The Science of Beauty* (New York: Anchor, 1999).

Bernhard Fink et al., "Visual Attention to Variation in Female Facial Skin Color Distribution," *Journal of Cosmetic Dermatology* 7 (2008): 155. This study tracked what men and women look at and judge to be attractive.

Jason M. Fletcher, "Beauty vs. Brains: Early Labor Market Outcomes of High School Graduates," *Economics Letters* 105 (2009): 321. This study showed that good-looking high school students do better than average and that there is a 3 percent to 5 percent "plainness penalty."

Daniel Hamermesh and Jeff Biddle, "Looks and the Labour Market," *American Economic Review* 84 (1994): 1174. One of Hamermesh's well-known studies on income and looks.

Daniel S. Hamermesh and Jason Abrevaya, "Beauty Is the Promise of Happiness," *European Economic Review* 64 (2013): 351. An international study on the direct and indirect impact of beauty on happiness.

David W. Johnston, "Physical Appearance and Wages: Do Blondes Have More Fun?," *Economics Letters* 108 (2010): 10. This study found that blondes make more money and marry wealthier men; it also discusses other studies regarding social value of blonde hair.

G. Kedia et al., "The Neural Correlates of Beauty Comparison," *Social Cognitive and Affective Neuroscience* 9 (2013): 681–88.

Douglas T. Kenrick and Sara E. Gutierres, "Contrast Effects and Judgments of Physical Attractiveness: When Beauty Becomes a Social Problem," *Journal of Personality and Social Psychology* 38 (1980): 131.

———, "Influence of Popular Erotica on Judgments of Strangers and Mates," *Journal of Experimental Social Psychology* 25 (1989): 159.

Geoff Kushnick, "Why Do the Karo Batak Prefer Women with Big Feet? Flexible Mate Preferences and the Notion That One Size Fits All," *Human Nature* 24, no. 3 (2013): 268.

D. G. Kwart et al., "Age and Beauty Are in the Eye of the Beholder," *Perception* 41 (2012): 925.

Anne E. Lincoln and Michael Patrick Allen, "Double Jeopardy in Hollywood: Age and Gender in the Careers of Film Actors, 1926–1999," *Sociological Forum* 19 (2004): 611. An example of a study that found a close link between perceptions of age and beauty.

Paul J. Matts and Bernhard Fink, "Chronic Sun Damage and the Perception of Age, Health and Attractiveness," *Photochemical and Photobiological Sciences* 9 (2010): 421. A review of evidence on how men perceive aging skin.

Ashley Mears, "Size Zero High-End Ethnic: Cultural Production and the Reproduction of Culture in Fashion Modeling," *Poetics* 38 (2010): 21.

Markus M. Mobius and Tanya S. Rosenblat, "Why Beauty Matters," *American Economic Review* 96 (2006): 222. Study highlights beauty premium.

Naci H. Mocan and Erdal Tekin, "Ugly Criminals," March 2006, IZA Discussion Paper No. 2048. This study for the German Institute for the Study of Labor (IZA) suggests that being "very attractive reduces a young adult's (ages 18–26) propensity for criminal activity."

Kate E. Mulgrew et al., "The Effect of Music Video Clips on Adolescent Boys' Body Image, Mood, and Schema Activation," *Journal of Youth and Adolescence* 43 (2013): 92–103.

M. J. Rantala et al., "Facial Attractiveness Is Related to Women's Cortisol and Body Fat, but Not with Immune Responsiveness," *Biology Letters* 9 (2013), doi: 10.1098 /rsbl.20130255. This study suggests that levels of stress may affect the attractiveness of women's faces.

Bradley Ruffle and Ze'ev Shtudiner, "Are Good-Looking People More Employable?," *Management Science*, Discussion Paper No. 10-06 (2010). This study includes data on good looks and employability, a big advantage for men but not for women. The authors speculate that "female jealousy of attractive women in the workplace is a primary reason for the punishment of attractive women."

Nadine Samson et al., "Visible Changes of Female Facial Skin Surface Topography in Relation to Age and Attractiveness Perception," *Journal of Cosmetic Dermatology* 9 (2010): 79. This study shows that even small, age-related changes to skin affect how women's faces are perceived by men.

Brent Scott and Timothy Judge, "Beauty, Personality, and Affect as Antecedents of Counterproductive Work Behavior Receipt Human Performance," *Human Performance* 26 (2013): 93. This study demonstrates that unattractive people are treated worse than attractive people.

Michelle Hannah Smirnova, "A Will to Youth: The Woman's Anti-Aging Elixir," *Social Science & Medicine* 75 (2012): 1236. This study of the advertising for antiaging products found that the consistent message implies that aging is a disease.

Society for Personality and Social Psychology, "Even Fact Will Not Change First Impressions," *ScienceDaily*, www.sciencedaily.com/releases/2014/02/140214111207 .htm.

Viren Swami et al., "More Than Just Skin Deep? Personality Information Influences Men's Ratings of the Attractiveness of Women's Body Sizes," *Journal of Social Psychology* 150 (2010): 628.

A. Tesser et al., "Some Affective Consequences of Social Comparison and Reflection Processes: The Pain and Pleasure of Being Close," *Journal of Personality and Social Psychology* 54 (1988): 49. A classic article on social comparison.

Marika Tiggemann and Janet Polivy, "Upward and Downward: Social Comparison Processing of Thin Idealized Media Images," *Psychology of Women Quarterly* 34 (2010): Q356. The authors write: "Results offer strong support to appearance social comparison as the mechanism by which idealized media images translate into body dissatisfaction for many women."

Takashi Tsukiura and Roberto Cabeza, "Shared Brain Activity for Aesthetic and Moral Judgments: Implications for the Beauty-Is-Good Stereotype," *SCAN* 6 (2010): 138. This study used brain-scan technology (fMRI) to show a connection between looks and perceptions of goodness.

Yuko Yamamiya et al., "Women's Exposure to Thin-and-Beautiful Media Images: Body Image Effects of Media-Ideal Internalization and Impact-Reduction Interventions," *Body Images* 2 (2005): 74.

CHAPTER 5: BEAUTY AND/OR HEALTH?

American Psychological Association, *Report of the APA Task Force on the Sexualization of Girls* (Washington, DC: American Psychological Association, 2010), www.apa .org/pi/women/programs/girls/report-full.pdf.

Jessica A. Boyce et al., "Positive Fantasies or Negative Contrasts: The Effect of Media Body Ideals on Restrained Eaters' Mood, Weight Satisfaction, and Food Intake," *Body Image* 10 (2013): 535.

S. A. Brown et al., "A Perceived Benefits and Barriers Scale for Strenuous Physical Activity in College Students," *American Journal of Health Promotion* 2 (2006): 137. This study explores why people exercise.

Joan C. Chrisler et al., "Suffering by Comparison: Twitter Users' Reactions to the Victoria's Secret Fashion Show," *Body Image* 10 (2013): 648.

Laura Hurd Clarke, "Older Women's Perceptions of Ideal Body Weights: The Tensions Between Health and Appearance Motivations for Weight Loss," *Ageing & Society* 22 (2002): 751.

John B. Dixon et al., "Motivation, Readiness to Change, and Weight Loss Following Adjustable Gastric Band Surgery," *Obesity* 17 (2009): 699. This study found that those who were motivated by appearance had better outcomes.

Marla E. Eisenberg et al., "Muscle-Enhancing Behaviors Among Adolescent Girls and Boys," *Pediatrics* 130 (2012): 1019. This study of steroid use concluded: "The use of muscle-enhancing behaviors is substantially higher than has been previously reported and is cause for concern."

Christopher J. Ferguson, "In the Eye of the Beholder: Thin-Ideal Media Affects Some, but Not Most, Viewers in a Meta-Analytic Review of Body Dissatisfaction in Women and Men," *Psychology of Popular Media Culture* 2 (2013): 20. An excellent meta-analysis and a reminder to not overinterpret the existing data.

Nicole M. Glenn et al., "Exploring Media Representations of Weight-Loss Surgery," *Qualitative Health Research* 23 (2013): 631.

S. Grabe et al., "The Role of the Media in Body Image Concerns Among Women: A Meta-Analysis of Experimental and Correlational Studies," *Psychology Bulletin* 134 (2008): 460.

David K. Ingledew and David Markland, "The Role of Motives in Exercise Participation," *Psychology & Health* 23 (2008): 807.

Andrew Johnson and Andy McSmith, "Children Say Being Famous Is Best Thing in World," *Independent* (UK), December 18, 2006, www.independent.co.uk/news/uk/this-britain/children-say-being-famous-is-best-thing-in-world-429000.html. A news report about a study highlighting the degree to which children value fame.

M. Kilpatrick et al., "College Students' Motivation for Physical Activity: Differentiating Men's and Women's Motives for Sport Participation and Exercise," *Journal of American College Health* 54 (2005): 87.

Margaret R. Laware and Chrisy Moutsatsos, "'For Skin That's Us, Authentically Us': Celebrity, Empowerment, and the Allure of Anti-Aging Advertisements," *Women's Studies in Communication* 36 (2013): 189. A study on the antiaging ads featuring Andie MacDowell and Diane Keaton.

John Maltby et al., "Intense-Personal Celebrity Worship and Body Image: Evidence of a Link Among Female Adolescents," *British Journal of Health Psychology* 10 (2005): 17.

Evelyn P. Meier and James Gray, "Facebook Photo Activity Associated with Body Image Disturbance in Adolescent Girls," *Cyberpsychology, Behavior, and Social Networking* 17 (2013): 199–206.

Kerry O'Brien et al., "Reasons for Wanting to Lose Weight: Different Strokes for Different Folks," *Eating Behaviors* 8 (2007): 132. The researchers studied why people diet, and one conclusion was that people who diet for the purpose of appearance are less happy.

M. Pankratow et al., "Effects of Reading Health and Appearance Exercise Magazine Articles on Perceptions of Attractiveness and Reasons for Exercise," *PLoS ONE* 8 (2013): e61894.

Erin Putterman and Wolfgang Linden, "Appearance Versus Health: Does the Reason for Dieting Affect Dieting Behavior?," *Journal of Behavioral Medicine* 27 (2004): 185.

Lindsey Tanner, "Steroid Use Much Higher Among Gay and Bi Teen Boys," Associated Press, February 3, 2014. This news report was on a study published in the journal *Pediatrics* in which the authors speculate about the desire for an ideal physique.

Pedro J. Teixeira et al., "Motivation, Self-Determination, and Long-Term Weight Control," *International Journal of Behavioral Nutrition and Physical Activity* 9 (2012): 1.

Lenny R. Vartanian et al., "Appearance vs. Health Motives for Exercise and for Weight Loss," *Psychology of Sport and Exercise* 13 (2012): 251–56.

Laura E. Willis and Silvia Knobloch-Westerwick, "Weighing Women Down: Messages on Weight Loss and Body Shaping in Editorial Content in Popular Women's Health and Fitness Magazines," *Health Communication* 29 (2013): 323–31. A study of over five thousand pages of women's magazines.

Ross D. Whitehead et al., "Appealing to Vanity: Could Potential Appearance Improvement Motivate Fruit and Vegetable Consumption?," *American Journal of Public Health* 102 (2012): 207. A commentary on the use of vanity as a public health tool and a review of relevant studies.

CHAPTER 6: DREAMS OF FAME AND FORTUNE

Emily Bishop et al., "Celebrity and Performance in the Hopes of Children," paper presented at the international colloquium Childhood and Cultures: Social and Human Sciences Perspectives, December 15–17, 2010, Paris, http://www.enfanceetcultures.culture.gouv.fr/actes/bishop_willis.pdf. This Australian study involved interviews with primary school kids.

Jake Halpern, "The Fame Survey," 2004, www.jakehalpern.com/famesurvey.php. A summary of a survey that included questions about being a celebrity assistant and how celebrity status is attained.

JWT Canada, *The American Dream in the Balance* (September 21, 2012), www.jwtcanada.ca/theamericandreaminthebalance. This marketing report notes that Americans increasingly view fame as part of the American dream.

Telegraph, "Children Would Rather Become Popstars Than Teachers or Lawyers," October 1, 2009, www.telegraph.co.uk/education/educationnews/6250626/Children-would-rather-become-popstars-than-teachers-or-lawyers.html.

CHAPTER 7: SO YOU WANT TO BE A STAR?

Moses Avalon, "What Are the Vegas Odds of Success on Today's Major Label Record Deal?," MosesAvalon.com, June 29, 2011, www.mosesavalon.com/what-are-the-vegas-odds-of-success-on-todays-major-label-record-deal/.

The BizParentz Foundation (www.bizparentz.org/home.html) provides statistics on child actors and "is a non-profit corporation providing education, advocacy, and charitable support to parents and children engaged in the entertainment industry." For statistics about more than twenty thousand child actors, see www.bizparentz.org/thebizness/pilotseason.html.

Scott Frank, "How Many Actors Are in L.A.? An Anthropologist Eyes the Entertain-
    ment Industry," *Hollywood Sapien*, July 5, 2012, http://hollywoodsapien.wordpress
    .com/about/. This article estimates that there are approximately 108,000 actors in
    Los Angeles.
————, "How Many Actors Are in New York? An Anthropologist Eyes the Entertain-
    ment Industry," *Hollywood Sapien*, December 13, 2012, http://hollywoodsapien
    .com/2012/12/13/how-many-actors-are-in-new-york/. The article estimates that
    New York has 28,963 professional actors in residence.
Bryden Haynes, "What Are the Odds of Succeeding Without a Record Deal?,"
    Music Think Tank, June 22, 2011, www.musicthinktank.com/blog/what-are
    -the-odds-of-succeeding-without-a-record-deal.html. This paper estimates the
    number of musicians in the United Kingdom who are "successful" without a
    record deal.
Alan B. Krueger, "Land of Hope and Dreams: Rock and Roll, Economics, and Rebuild-
    ing the Middle Class," speech, White House, June 12, 2013, www.whitehouse
    .gov/sites/default/files/docs/hope_and_dreams_-_final.pdf. This is an economic
    analysis of the music industry, with comments on luck.
Office of Research and Analysis, National Endowment for the Arts, *Artist Unemploy-
    ment Rates for 2008 and 2009* (Washington, DC, January 2010), http://arts.gov
    /sites/default/files/97-update.pdf. The bulletin states: "Unemployment rates for
    actors tend to be the highest among all artist occupations."
Nordicity, *Sound Analysis: An Examination of the Canadian Independent Music Indus-
    try*, February 2013, www.nordicity.com/media/201336fjtnrdeunp.pdf. A report
    prepared for the Canadian Independent Music Association.
Zachary Pincus-Roth, "The Feasibility of Living in Manhattan on a Chorus Member's
    Salary," *Playbill*, August 31, 2007, www.playbill.com/features/article/print/110695
    .html. Estimates that 88 percent of card-holding actors are unemployed in New
    York City at any one time.
William J. Price, "What Are the Odds of Becoming a Professional Athlete?," United
    States Sports Academy, *Sports Digest*, http://thesportdigest.com/archive/article
    /what-are-odds-becoming-professional-athlete.html. Statistics on the chances of
    making it as a professional athlete. The author looks at high school seniors for his
    data set.
PRLog, "Over Half of Young People Want to Be Famous," February 17, 2010, www
    .prlog.org/10536256-over-half-of-young-people-want-to-be-famous.html.
Michael Simkins, "When the Going Gets Tough," op-ed, *Guardian* (UK), May 9,
    2009, www.guardian.co.uk/stage/2009/may/09/tips-surviving-acting-industry.
    Highlights how tough it is to find work as an actor. Simkins writes: "The old
    maxim still holds true: if you can think of any other career that would give you
    the same sense of satisfaction or peace of mind, do that instead. You'll get little of
    either as an actor."
Randy Turner, "Parents Who Can Afford It Scramble to Get Kids into Elite Hockey
    Programs," *Winnipeg Free Press*, February 2, 2013, www.winnipegfreepress.com
    /opinion/fyi/spring-fever-189487451.html. This article quotes parents' expecta-
    tions regarding making it as a player in the National Hockey League.

CHAPTER 8: CELEBRITY DREAMS AND COGNITIVE BIASES

Ozgun Atasoy, "You Are Less Beautiful Than You Think," *Scientific American*, May 21, 2013, www.scientificamerican.com/article.cfm?id=you-are-less-beautiful-than -you-think. Summarizes relevant data on beauty.

Orville Gilbert Brim, interview, University of Michigan Press website, 2009, www .press.umich.edu/pdf/9780472070701_qa.pdf. Brim suggests that there are twenty thousand "fame" slots for about four million fame seekers.

———, *Look at Me! The Fame Motive from Childhood to Death* (Ann Arbor: University of Michigan Press, 2009).

Jonathon D. Brown, "Understanding the Better Than Average Effect: Motives (Still) Matter," *Personality and Social Psychology Bulletin* 38 (2012): 209.

T. Chamorro-Premuzic et al., "Assessing Pupils' Intelligence through Self, Parental, and Teacher Estimates," *Educational Psychology* 29 (2009): 83.

Nicholas Epley and David Dunning, "Feeling 'Holier Than Thou': Are Self-Serving Assessments Produced by Errors in Self- or Social Prediction?," *Journal of Personality and Social Psychology* 79 (2000): 861. This study showed that people think they are more selfless, kind, and generous than others.

Nicholas Epley and Erin Whitchurch, "Mirror, Mirror on the Wall: Enhancement in Self-Recognition," *Personality and Social Psychology Bulletin* 34 (2008): 1159.

Bruno S. Frey and Beat Heggli, "An Ipsative Theory of Business Behaviour," *Journal of Economic Psychology* 10, no. 1 (1989). This study notes unrealistic optimism.

Dominic D. P. Johnson, and James H. Fowler, "The Evolution of Overconfidence," *Nature* 477 (2011): 317.

Verena Jung et al., "Antecedents of Attitudes Towards Risky Career Choices," EBS Business School Research Paper No. 12–10, 2012, http://ssrn.com/abstract= 2185429 or http://dx.doi.org/10.2139/ssrn.2185429.

———, "What Shapes Young Elite Athletes' Perception of Chances in an Environment of Great Uncertainty?," CREMA Working Paper Series 2012–14, Center for Research in Economics, Management and the Arts, Switzerland, http://external -apps.qut.edu.au/business/documents/discussionPapers/2012/WP292.pdf. This study demonstrates the unrealistic optimism among German soccer players. It also has a nice summary of relevant literature and includes a quote from Adam Smith.

S. B. Kårstad et al., "What Do Parents Know About Their Children's Comprehension of Emotions? Accuracy of Parental Estimates in a Community Sample of Pre-Schoolers," *Child: Care, Health and Development* 40 (2013): 346–53.

James C. Kaufman et al., "The *American Idol* Effect: Are Students Good Judges of Their Creativity Across Domains?," *Empirical Studies of the Arts* 28 (2010): 3. An interesting study of fourth-grade students' ability to assess their own talents.

Heather C. Lench et al., "My Child Is Better Than Average: The Extension and Restriction of Unrealistic Optimism," *Journal of Applied Social Psychology* 36 (2006): 2963. An example of a study that demonstrated how parents view their kids' abilities.

Valerie F. Reyna and Charles J. Brainerd, "Numeracy, Ratio Bias, and Denominator Neglect in Judgments of Risk and Probability," *Learning and Individual Differences* 18 (2008): 89.

Punit Shah, "Toward a Neurobiology of Unrealistic Optimism," *Frontiers in Psychology* 3 (2012): 1. A nice review of the science behind optimistic bias. Shah writes: "Optimism bias is a robust phenomenon with a neurobiological basis."

Tali Sharot et al., "How Unrealistic Optimism Is Maintained in the Face of Reality," *Nature Neuroscience* 14 (2011): 1475. A neuroscience study on biological basis of optimistic bias.

Cass R. Sunstein, "Probability Neglect: Emotions, Worst Cases, and Law," *Yale Law Journal* 112 (2003): 61.

William von Hippel and Robert Trivers, "The Evolution and Psychology of Self-Deception," *Behavioral and Brain Sciences* 34 (2011): 1.

N. D. Weinstein, "Unrealistic Optimism About Future Life Events," *Journal of Personality and Social Psychology* 39 (1980): 806. One of the best-known papers exploring the phenomenon of unrealistic optimism.

CHAPTER 9: SIMON COWELL AND SOCIAL PRESSURE

Eric Flack, "Talent Search Under Fire for Use of Disney Name," *Wave 3 News*, June 5, 2012, www.wave3.com/story/18708180/talent-search-uses-disney-name-not-really-for-disney. One of many stories highlighting acting scams aimed at kids.

Marvin Joseph, "Kids Try On Model Behavior," *Washington Post*, April 5, 2013, www.highbeam.com/doc/1P2-34482273.html.

Y. T. Uhls and P. M. Greenfield, "The Rise of Fame: An Historical Content Analysis," *Cyberpsychology: Journal of Psychosocial Research on Cyberspace* 5, no. 1 (2011). Study analyzed representation of fame in popular media.

———, "The Value of Fame: Preadolescent Perceptions of Popular Media and Their Relationship to Future Aspirations," *Developmental Psychology* 48 (2011): 315. Noted the degree to which fame is a dominant value and goal.

CHAPTER 10: LUCK AND TEN THOUSAND HOURS

BBC News Online, "Celebrity Culture 'Harms Pupils,'" *BBC*, March 14, 2008, http://news.bbc.co.uk/1/hi/education/7296306.stm. Reports on UK teachers' perspectives on students' desire for fame.

David J. Berri and Brian Burke, "Measuring Productivity of NFL Players," in *The Economics of the National Football League: The State of the Art*, ed. Kevin G. Quinn (New York: Springer, 2012). Emphasizes the challenges and complexities associated with measuring productivity.

D. Berri and R. Simmons, "Catching a Draft: On the Process of Selecting Quarterbacks in the National Football League Amateur Draft," *Journal of Productivity Analysis* 35 (2009): 37.

Malcolm Gladwell, *Outliers: The Story of Success* (New York: Little, Brown, 2008).

David (Zach) Hambrick et al., "Deliberate Practice: Is That All It Takes to Become an Expert?," *Intelligence* 45 (2013): 34–45.

D. J. Koz et al., "Accuracy of Professional Sports Drafts in Predicting Career Potential," *Scandinavian Journal of Medicine & Science in Sports* 22 (2012): e64. This study "highlight[s] the challenges of accurately evaluating amateur talent."

Matthew Salganik and Duncan Watts, "Leading the Herd Astray: An Experimental Study of Self-Fulfilling Prophecies in an Artificial Cultural Market," *Social Psychology* 71 (2008): Q338. Showed the randomness of getting a hit song. It was also mentioned in Alan B. Krueger, "Land of Hope and Dreams," above.

Ross Tucker and Malcolm Collins, "What Makes Champions? A Review of the Relative Contribution of Genes and Training to Sporting Success," *British Journal of Sports Medicine* 46 (2012): 555.

CHAPTER 11: A LONELY, HEALTH-DESTROYING GRIND?

Katherine Marie Jacobs Bao, "Aspirations and Well-Being: When Are High Aspirations Harmful?," PhD diss., University of California, Riverside, 2013, www .escholarship.org/uc/item/2mb048sx?query=%22aspirations%20and%20well -being%22.

D. R. Beike et al., "What We Regret Most Are Lost Opportunities: A Theory of Regret Intensity," *Personality and Social Psychology Bulletin* 35 (2008): 385.

Mark A. Bellis et al., "Dying to Be Famous: Retrospective Cohort Study of Rock and Pop Star Mortality and Its Association with Adverse Childhood Experiences," *BMJ Open* (2012): e002089, doi:10.1136/bmjopen-2012-002089.

———, "Elvis to Eminem: Quantifying the Price of Fame Through Early Mortality of European and North American Rock and Pop Stars," *Journal of Epidemiological Community Health* 61 (2007): 896. This study found that fame increased mortality risk by more than 1.7 times.

Philip Brickman et al., "Lottery Winners and Accident Victims: Is Happiness Relative?," *Journal of Personality and Social Psychology* 36 (1978): 917.

E. Brummelman et al., "My Child Redeems My Broken Dreams: On Parents Transferring Their Unfulfilled Ambitions onto Their Child," *PLoS ONE* 8 (2013): e65360.

J. J. Connor et al., "Would They Dope? Revisiting the Goldman Dilemma," *British Journal of Sports Medicine* 47 (2012): 697. A study on the number of people in the general population who would take performance-enhancing drugs even if it shortened their life.

C. R. Epstein and R. J. Epstein, "Death in *The New York Times*: The Price of Fame Is a Faster Flame," *QJM [Quarterly Journal of Medicine]* 106 (2013): 517.

Daniel Gilbert, *Stumbling on Happiness* (New York: Random House, 2006).

Joshua Halberstam, "Fame," *American Philosophical Quarterly* 21 (January 1984): Q93. Halberstam writes: "Those who desire fame as a source of pleasure believe that being famous will somehow or other improve their present lives."

Xu Han et al., "The Effect of Winning an Oscar Award on Survival: Correcting for Healthy Performer Survivor Bias with a Rank Preserving Structural Accelerated Failure Time Model," *Annals of Applied Statistics* 5 (2011): 746. Han writes: "There is not strong evidence that winning an Oscar increases life expectancy." The paper also provides a nice review of literature.

J. Holt-Lunstad et al., "Social Relationships and Mortality Risk: A Meta-Analytic Review," *PLoS Medicine* 7 (2010): e1000316.

James House et al., "Social Relationships and Health," *Science* 241 (1988): 540. An often-referenced paper on the value of relationships to health.

Tim Kasser, "Further Examining the American Dream: Differential Correlates of Intrinsic and Extrinsic Goals," *Personality and Social Psychology Bulletin* 22 (1996): 280. An often-cited paper on the impact of intrinsic and extrinsic goals on well-being.

John Maltby, "An Interest in Fame: Confirming the Measurement and Empirical Conceptualization of Fame Interest," *British Journal of Psychology* 101 (2010): 411. A good analysis of the dimensions of the fame interest. Also, it refers to UK surveys about interest in fame, including a BBC story.

John Maltby et al., "Implicit Theories of a Desire for Fame," *British Journal of Psychology* 99 (2008): 279. Outlines key reasons people seek fame, including "social access" and deriving meaning by comparison to others.

Thomas Niederkrotenthaler et al., "Changes in Suicide Rates Following Media Reports on Celebrity Suicide: A Meta-Analysis," *Journal of Epidemiology and Community Health* 66 (2012): 1037. Suicide rates increase with reports of celebrity suicides.

D. Rockwell and D. C. Giles, "Being a Celebrity: A Phenomenology of Fame," *Journal of Phenomenological Psychology* 40 (2009): 178.

Kennon M. Sheldon et al., "Extrinsic Value Orientation and Affective Forecasting: Overestimating the Rewards, Underestimating the Costs," *Journal of Personality* 78 (2010): 149. The authors write: "It appears that some people overestimate the emotional benefits of achieving extrinsic goals, to their potential detriment."

K. M. Sheldon and S. Lyubomirsky, "The Challenge of Staying Happier: Testing the Hedonic Adaptation Prevention Model," *Personality and Social Psychology Bulletin* 38 (2012): 670. The impact of aspiration on levels of happiness.

Jacqueline Stenson, "Kids on Steroids Willing to Risk It All for Success," *NBC News*, March 3, 2008, www.nbcnews.com/id/22984780/. Reviews steroids statistics.

John Tierney, "From Tinseltown to Splitsville: Just Do the Math," *New York Times*, September 19, 2006, www.nytimes.com/2006/09/19/opinion/19tierney.html?_r=1&scp=4&sq=Garth+Sundem&st=nyt. The "formula" for predicting how long a celebrity marriage will last (not long).

———, "Refining the Formula That Predicts Celebrity Marriages' Doom," *New York Times*, March 12, 2012, www.nytimes.com/2012/03/13/science/a-refined-formula-to-predict-doom-in-celebrity-marriages.html?pagewanted=1&_r=1&. An update on the divorce formula.

Pablo S. Torre, "How (and Why) Athletes Go Broke," *Sports Illustrated*, March 23, 2009, http://www.si.com/vault/2009/03/23/105789480/how-and-why-athletes-go-broke.

Debra Umberson et al., "You Make Me Sick: Marital Quality and Health over the Life Course," *Journal of Health and Social Behavior* 47, no. 1 (2006).

Jie Zhang et al., "Psychological Strains Found in the Suicides of 72 Celebrities," *Journal of Affective Disorders* 149 (2013): 230. Explores the themes present in celebrity suicides. The authors used this method to explore their theory of "strain" in the context of suicide.

CONCLUSION: THE DREAM CRUSHER?

Krystal Beamon and Patricia A. Bell, "'Going Pro': The Deferential Effects of High Aspirations for a Professional Sports Career on African-American Student Athletes and White Student Athletes," *Race and Society* 5 (2002): 179–91.

Consumer Federation of America, "How Americans View Personal Wealth vs. How Financial Planners View This Wealth," January 2006, http://www.consumerfed .org/pdfs/Financial_Planners_Study011006.pdf. This survey found that people believe a lottery is a practical way to accumulate wealth.

Nick Couldry and Tim Markham, "Celebrity Culture and Public Connection: Bridge or Chasm?," *International Journal of Cultural Studies* 10 (2007): 403.

Economic Mobility Project, *Pursuing the American Dream: Economic Mobility Across Generations* (Washington, DC: Pew Charitable Trusts, July 2012), http://www .pewtrusts.org/en/research-and-analysis/reports/0001/01/01/pursuing-the -american-dream.

Howard Steven Friedman, "The American Myth of Social Mobility," *Huffington Post*, July 16, 2012, www.huffingtonpost.com/howard-steven-friedman/class-mobility _b_1676931.html. This article contains the quote about America as the land of opportunity.

Bobcat Goldthwait, "Don't Be Afraid to Quit, Success Is Overrated," 2009 commencement speech at Hampshire College, Amherst, MA, posted May 22, 2012, http://boingboing.net/2012/05/22/bobcat-goldthwaite-commencemen.html.

John Helliwell, Richard Layard, and Jeffrey Sachs, eds., *World Happiness Report 2013* (New York: UN Sustainable Development Solutions Network, 2013). There are a variety of other happiness reports. One was produced by the UN's Organisation for Economic Co-operation and Development (it placed Australia at the top); see http://www.oecdbetterlifeindex.org/topics/life-satisfaction/; another, produced by the Legatum Institute, is the *Prosperity Index*, and in 2013 it placed Norway, Switzerland, and Canada at the top (www.prosperity.com/#!/?aspxerrorpath= %2Frankings.aspx). I selected the UN ranking as it seemed the most comprehensive and focused on the concept of happiness.

Organisation for Economic Co-operation and Development, *A Family Affair: Intergenerational Social Mobility Across OECD Countries* (OECD, 2010), www.oecd .org/centrodemexico/medios/44582910.pdf.

———, *PISA 2012 Results* (OECD, 2013), www.oecd.org/pisa/keyfindings/pisa-2012 -results-overview.pdf. This ranking of education systems shows relative poor performance of the United States and United Kingdom.

Estrella Romero et al., "Life Aspirations, Personality Traits and Subjective Well-Being in a Spanish Sample," *European Journal of Personality* 26, no. 1 (2012): 45–55. This study showed the well-being associated with striving for intrinsic rewards.

Karen Sternheimer, *Celebrity Culture and the American Dream: Stardom and Social Mobility* (New York: Routledge, 2013).

Jean M. Twenge, "The Evidence for Generation Me and Against Generation We," *Emerging Adulthood* 1 (2013): 11–16.

Jean M. Twenge and Jeffrey Arnett, "A Back and Forth About Narcissism," discussion, *New York Times*, August 5, 2013, http://www.nytimes.com/2013/08/06/science/a-back-and-forth-about-narcissism.html?_r=0.

Jean M. Twenge and W. Keith Campbell, *The Narcissism Epidemic: Living in the Age of Entitlement* (New York: Free Press, 2009).

Joe Weisenthal, "Here's the New Ranking of Top Countries in Reading, Science, and Math," *Business Insider*, December 3, 2013, http://www.businessinsider.com/pisa-rankings-2013-12. A report on the OECD rankings.

INDEX